EATING FOR
BETTER HEALTH

HOW DIET CAN HELP YOU FIGHT AND PREVENT MANY
COMMON HEALTH PROBLEMS

PROFESSOR JANE PLANT CBE
AND GILL TIDEY

Foreword by
Dr Michael Dixon OBE

2 4 6 8 10 9 7 5 3 1

Published in 2010 by Virgin Books, an imprint of Ebury Publishing
A Random House Group Company

Address

A CIP

The Ran
[FSC], th
that are

ISBN 9780753519493

To buy books by your favourite authors and register for offers visit
www.rbooks.co.uk

Typeset by TW Typesetting, Plymouth, Devon
Printed and bound in the UK by CPI Bookmarque, Croydon CR0 4TD

Contents

Authors' Note

The diagnosis and treatment of medical conditions is a responsibility shared between you and your medical advisors. All diets should begin with a medical checkup to make certain that no special health problems exist and to confirm that there are no medical reasons why you should not undertake a change of diet.

Acknowledgements

Jane and Gill would like to thank their husbands, Peter Simpson and David Falvey, for their encouragement, support and practical help with the book. They also acknowledge the help of Jane's son Tom, a doctor, for critically reviewing the medical sections of the book. Dr Henry Haslam helped with the revision of this new edition. Dr Sylvia Haslam made a helpful contribution to the section on ME/CFS.

For more information about Jane and how to contact her, please see www.janeplant.com.

Foreword

This is a book that you will find hard to put down. It is not just fascinating and informative: it is also intensely practical. For many, it may well be a life saver. Indeed, it should probably be compulsory reading for every adult and in every household. For the uninitiated, much of its content will be new and inspirational, but even the most experienced doctor and therapist will find something new here.

'We are what we eat' has become a cliché, but 'healthy eating' for much of the British population is an oxymoron. It is predicted that in fifteen years' time almost half of the adult population will be obese. It is also predicted that our children will die younger than ourselves, simply because of obesity. Yet the UK spends less on its food, in proportion to its gross domestic product, than any other developed country. Diabetes, heart disease, cancer and a whole range of other chronic diseases are, in many cases, the result of a poor diet and, in an equal number, can be remedied by getting our diet right. Yet for the majority it is almost a question of 'we don't care what we eat'. This book illustrates wonderfully why we should care and, more importantly, shows us exactly how we can improve our health and resistance to disease in clear and practical ways.

The problems that this book seeks to solve go beyond the health and well-being of each of us as individuals, going to the heart of issues of public health and affordability of the health service. Getting our diet right costs very little when compared with the expense of treatment. The cost of pills, technology and hospital care to overcome the problems of bad diet will soon make every health service unaffordable. If we help ourselves and each other by eating more healthily, exercising more and living more fulfilling lives then we will be able to afford expensive technology for when it is appropriate and necessary. A good diet is not a panacea, but it is something that we can adopt fairly easily with a little bit of determination.

It is always flattering to be asked to write a foreword to a book. The downside too often is that you also have to read it! Not so this book. Once I opened it, I found it difficult to stop reading. It is much more than simply a 'good read', however. It is packed with the best evidence that we have on healthy eating. Academics may quibble about the weight of evidence for some of the assertions, but they will be missing the point. The point is that in real life we have to make the best use of the best available evidence, and anyone taking advice from this book will be 90 per cent down the route towards better eating and health. They will also have a far better understanding of food itself and how different foods contribute to different aspects of our health. This may lead to a greater interest in and connection with the different foods and how and where they are grown. For too many of us, food is simply a fuel. Fats, carbohydrates and proteins are just the diesel, leaded and unleaded petrol that keep us going. In reality, we should regard our eating habits as a complex and wonderful mixture of art and science. We should appreciate food's complexity and also its power to heal and improve health. By being both practical and interesting and with a vast range of recipes to illustrate its lessons, this book should create a new generation of healthy-eating advocates, who will influence and interest those around them and improve their health and well-being.

As a GP, I will be recommending this book to my patients, ensuring that we have several copies in our patients' library, and I shall take a copy home to try and influence those younger members of my family who think that they will live for ever and assume that healthy eating is just for health-conscious adults. So by all means use this book as a practical set of tips and recipes to guide your own path to better health, but do not be afraid to be an evangelist and pass the word on to those who might otherwise suffer. Congratulations to both authors on a courageous, inspiring and brilliant book.

Dr Michael Dixon OBE MA (Hons, Oxon) Psychology and Philosophy
MB BS LRCP DRCOG MRCGP FRCGP

Medical Director, Prince's Foundation for Integrated Health
Chair, NHS Alliance
Visiting Professor, The University of Westminster
Honorary Senior Fellow in the School of Public Policy, University of
    Birmingham
Honorary Senior Lecturer in Integrated Health at Peninsula Medical School

Introduction

WELCOME

As with all our books published since *Your Life in Your Hands* was first launched in June 2000, this book has been written in response to many requests from our readers. Jane's international bestseller *Your Life in Your Hands* describes her experience of breast cancer, which recurred four times after her initial mastectomy and involved her in four further operations, thirty-five radiotherapy treatments, irradiation of her ovaries to induce menopause, and twelve chemotherapy treatments. The book tells how she used her scientific knowledge and experience of working in China to identify dairy produce as the principal factor promoting her breast cancer. Within five weeks of eliminating all dairy produce from her otherwise healthy diet and lifestyle, a large secondary tumour in her neck had totally disappeared, and she has now been free of cancer for sixteen years. Following the success of this book, Jane teamed up with Gill to write *The Plant Programme*, which provides a dietary regime, with lots of delicious recipes to help breast-cancer and prostate-cancer sufferers.

This book is based on the many communications we have received about how, as well as helping to overcome cancer, our diet has helped cancer sufferers' health in so many other ways. For example, many have told us that their blood pressure has fallen, their heart condition has improved and their type-2 diabetes has disappeared. Others have reported that their mood has lightened and they have become more positive, while others who have suffered for years from bowel problems or cystitis or even thrush say these problems no longer trouble them.

Many, many people tell us how their skin has improved. We were struck by a comment made by a young publicist provided by Virgin Books to go with us to the talks we gave in the early days. After accompanying us to two or three of these events, which are always followed by a queue of people wanting to talk to us, the young woman said, 'There is something that puzzles me – I can understand that people want to talk to you about their illness, I can understand why they want you to sign their books, but why do so many people roll up their sleeves and show you their perfectly healthy arms?' It took a few minutes before we realised the answer – 'Oh, they are showing us that their psoriasis or eczema has gone,' we replied. Indeed, many people tell us how their skin, hair, nails and body shape have improved greatly by following our programme. When we talk to breast-cancer support groups and meet people who initially contacted us when they were desperate, we are always impressed by how well those following our regime look.

The Plant Programme was written primarily with cancer sufferers in mind. *Eating for Better Health* contains over 150 new recipes, based on the same dietary principles but for a much wider range of chronic diseases. We describe many of the chronic conditions that are acknowledged to be related to a poor diet and that are presently taking an enormous toll on the health, social and financial welfare of Western industrialised countries and, increasingly, the developing world. We explain how diet and different foods can help to prevent and treat conditions ranging from cardiovascular disease to diabetes and from anxiety and depression to bone disease. We know personally of people who have found our diet helpful for all of the conditions described in the book. In some cases, the book is based on personal experience: for example, Jane has experienced bouts of anxiety and depression.

The book begins by explaining the principles of our approach. We then discuss systematically which foods to eat and which to avoid, using ten easy-to-follow food factors. This is followed by a description of numerous illnesses and conditions in which the Western diet is strongly implicated as one of the major causative factors, and we emphasise the foods that are particularly important for each condition. The second part of the book is a great cookbook, based on our four principles:

- The food is healthy and nutritious.
- The recipes are simple and easy to follow.

2

- The whole way of cooking is practical and the recipes are mostly inexpensive and quick to make.
- The dishes are tempting and delicious.

We hope to persuade you to cook freshly made meals rather than rely on convenience and processed food.

Within a few weeks of following the Plant Programme diet you will probably look and feel much better and wonder how your body managed to cope with your old eating habits. Most obese and overweight people who follow our plan lose weight and are able to sustain their trimmer shape over the longer term. Hair, eyes and skin, and even nails, usually improve. We hope that this book will help many people to prevent or treat their chronic illnesses. From all the feedback we have received we know you will be amazed at just how delicious our recipes are.

Remember, there is nothing strange or faddish about our approach. Unlike many modern fad diets, ours is mainly based on the traditional Chinese diet that has evolved over a period of at least 4,500 years, although we have modified it to suit Western tastes. The result is a distinctive East-meets-West style of food, influenced particularly by Chinese and Mediterranean cooking.

So – enjoy eating our food, at the same time as improving your health.
Jane and Gill

WHAT IS THE PROBLEM?

At the present time North America, Europe and Australia are facing an epidemic of chronic diseases that is now sweeping across the world in the wake of the Western diet.[1] It has been estimated, for example, that almost half of all Americans will suffer from cancer, which has recently overtaken heart disease as the biggest killer in America. The health and social services of these countries are under unprecedented pressure to cope, and vast amounts of money are being spent on coronary bypass operations, hip, knee and other joint replacements and a range of pills and potions, often with their own serious side-effects, administered by hard-

---

[1] Chronic diseases as used here include degenerative diseases such as diabetes, cardiovascular diseases, depression and osteoporosis, but not infectious diseases such as tuberculosis and HIV/AIDS.

pressed medical professionals. In the UK, the annual spend on health care now exceeds £100 billion and by 2007 the equivalent spend in the US was $2.26 trillion. There is increasingly a sense among patients and health professionals that prevention really is better than cure. As well as being better for patients' wellbeing, it can be more effective and much less expensive than waiting for disease to occur and then attempting to treat it – as is currently the main focus of most national health-care systems.

Many people are trying to help cure themselves, often using unsuitable alternative medicine picked up in a health-food shop, or following fad diets which may be expensive, have no effect at all or even make things worse. A widely held view is that many common health problems relate to an ageing population, but the conditions are affecting younger and younger people and spreading throughout the developing world as they follow the spread of the Western fast-food–junk-food culture.

Let us take obesity as one example of a diet-related disease that is also a serious condition underlying many other increasingly common diseases. Obesity continues to increase dramatically. During the late 1990s, for example, nearly one-third of all adult Americans were classified as obese by a national health and nutrition survey, and 64 per cent of the adult population were found to be overweight. Obesity levels have also risen sharply in Australia, Canada and Europe. The rise in obesity has been accompanied by a dramatic increase in cardiovascular disease and also an increase in diabetes, arthritis and some cancers. Trends in the national health status of developing countries undergoing rapid economic growth indicate a decrease in protein deficiency but a marked rise in obesity, especially in urban areas. For example, in urban areas in South Africa 56 per cent of women are now clinically obese and in urban areas in Brazil there has been more than a 100 per cent increase in this condition in the last twenty years.

There is little doubt that the increase in obesity reflects poor diet. In much of Europe and North America, fat and sugar now account for more than half the calorie intake, and refined carbohydrate has largely replaced whole-grained foods. In the USA 98 per cent of wheat is now refined. The UK diet is also dominated by refined wheat and animal produce such as meat and dairy, with much less fruit, vegetables and fish eaten now than during the Second World War. Most dramatic of all has been the change in the amount of fast and convenience foods consumed. The average person now eats more than 4kg (8lb) of food additives a year.

A few facts from the World Heart Federation:

- In the USA, sales of salty snacks such as crisps and salted peanuts increased by 6 per cent between 1995 and 1999. Potato crisps are the first choice for snacks for about 80 per cent of American adults and about 75 per cent of children.
- Americans are now consuming twice as many fizzy drinks as they did 25 years ago.
- Americans spend about half of their food budget on meals eaten out, which are generally higher in bad fats (see table on dietary fats on page 39) and lower in essential micronutrients than food prepared at home.

Our view is that many of the increasingly common chronic diseases are caused by poor diet, which contains large amounts of damaging fatty, salty, sugary and generally over-refined processed foods that are high in man-made chemicals. The typical Western diet also contains too much animal produce in relation to vegetable foods. A recent survey in the UK involving more than 37,000 people compared consumption of certain specific food groups with general wellbeing. It demonstrated that the food and drink in the typical UK diet, including, as it does, sugar-based snacks, refined food, red meat, tea and coffee, salt and dairy produce, appeared to have negative associations with health, with a direct relationship between how much is eaten and the severity of symptoms.

Our programme is not aimed simply at weight loss while ignoring other possible adverse health effects. It is aimed at all-round good health, and it should help to lead to the healthy body condition that is right for you.

We emphasise that our programme should be used to complement, not replace, conventional medicine. We recommend that all conditions should be diagnosed by medical professionals and changes to diet discussed with them.

PART ONE – FOOD AND HEALTH

The Principles of the Plant Programme

Our programme is based on the use of unprocessed foods produced as healthily as possible and with a high proportion of vegetable foods, including fruit, vegetables, herbs and spices, seeds, nuts and pulses. Living foods still contain their food enzymes – enzymes that are destroyed by the prolonged storage, processing and cooking procedures that are involved in the production of what we call 'fossil' foods. The programme is also aimed at obtaining the best proportions and the right types of proteins, fats, carbohydrates, vitamins, minerals and health-protective plant chemicals in the diet.

We advise on how to achieve the optimum acid–alkali balance in the body and show how to minimise the need to take man-made vitamin or mineral supplements, which have been implicated in causing ill health. The advantages of organically produced food are described, with reference to the standards of the Soil Association, which is the UK's leading campaigning and certification organisation for organic food and farming.

The main problem with the modern industrialised Western diet is that it includes:

- Foods that are innately bad for health, such as dairy (see also our books *Your Life in Your Hands*, *Prostate Cancer* and *Osteoporosis*), the meat of factory-reared livestock and other foods high in saturated fats, hormones, growth factors and other harmful biologically active substances. Consuming such food also increases the risk of exposure to dangerous pathogens such as *E. coli* (0157), salmonella and listeria, which are responsible for an increasing number of serious cases of food poisoning and associated illness. For some people, eating gluten-rich foods such as wheat and related cereal products can cause health problems.
- Food and drink that contain high concentrations of man-made chemicals. For example, vegetables can contain pesticides and soil conditioners like acrylamide, and animal products can have

residues of veterinary medicines such as antibiotics and anti-parasitic drugs. More than four hundred specific chemical compounds are currently registered for use as insecticides in the USA, for example. These agrochemical pollutants are in addition to general environmental pollutants, ranging from chemicals used in plastics and pharmaceuticals to chemical residues from industrial processes and energy generation. All of these chemicals can be damaging to physical and/or mental well-being.

• Foods that are over-refined and over-processed so that essential nutrients are removed, leaving behind only empty calories. Additives such as antioxidants, preservatives, emulsifiers, food colorants and flavouring agents, including sweeteners, are frequently incorporated in such products during food processing and manufacture. In the European Union more than 1,500 food additives are allowed. These range from aspartame E951, a man-made sweetener that has been suggested to be connected to behavioural and other health problems, to tartrazine E102, a yellow colorant suggested to cause hyperactivity in children. These substances are increasingly used in fast, convenience and processed foods to enhance taste, texture, consistency, colour or 'mouth feel' and to give food longer shelf life so that it has frequently been 'dead' for a long time before we eat it – which is why we call it 'fossil food'.

Even food containers from fast-food outlets were, until recently, impregnated with a grease-proofing chemical now known to accumulate in the human blood and be associated with bladder cancer. Other chemicals leached from plastic wrappings have been shown to have endocrine-disrupting (hormone-disrupting) properties with implications for reproductive cancers (breast, ovarian, womb, prostate and testicular).

SOME PROBLEMS WITH CURRENT FAD AND 'HEALTHY' DIETS

HIGH-PROTEIN, LOW-CARBOHYDRATE DIET

The high-protein, low-carbohydrate diet, which continues to be extremely popular for weight loss, is highly controversial, as it can produce a state of ketosis whereby the body burns only stored fat for fuel because of the absence of carbohydrates. Vital electrolytes, especially potassium, can be lowered dangerously, leading to an increased risk of irregular heartbeat (heart arrhythmia) and heart attacks. People following such diets, even in the short term, tend to suffer from constipation (animal produce contains no fibre) and other digestive problems, mood swings, depression and headaches. Carried to excess, such diets will leach the bones, muscle and other tissues because of the acid generated by the consumption of large amounts of animal protein (see table on pages 28–29). Moreover, the rapid initial loss of weight noted by some people who try such diets is more likely to be due to a reduction of bone density and body protein than to loss of fat, because the former have much higher densities (fat floats on water whereas muscle meat sinks, and certainly bone does).

Let us give you just two examples of the many people we have met who are followers of this type of diet. The first was a woman who we thought was at least 60 years old but who turned out to be 46 and who had been on such a diet for 2½ years. She had lost some weight, but admitted that her waist measurement was little changed. In addition, she was still seriously obese, her breath smelled, she had thinning hair and acne and complained that her back and all her joints ached so much she could hardly sleep. Compare this with a man who had followed our diet for three years. He is 68 years old but looks much younger, and has reduced his waist measurement by about four inches. He had osteoarthritis in both hip joints, both knees, and the lower back but, although he still has a limp on one side caused by residual damage in one hip, he now has no pain and has complete flexibility in all his other joints.

The second example was a young man in his early 20s, looking frail and at least twenty years older than his age, who had had Crohn's disease for much of his life. Listening to him, there seemed to have been a marked deterioration in his condition since he took up the high-protein low-carbohydrate diet. He had been treated with steroids for Crohn's disease, which had caused some bone thinning – osteoporosis – but after starting the high-protein low-carbohydrate diet this had become so severe that he was now being treated with yet another drug to try to arrest this condition.

Compare this with a young woman who, when we first met her, had osteoporosis caused by anorexia, accompanied by severe acne. At the time, all she was consuming was milk, to which a powdered food supplement was added. She took control by following our programme and now has normal bone density, a slim figure but within the normal range, and her acne has cleared totally.

There are many people who, after reading our books, have told us that they attribute their present health problems, ranging from cancer to constipation and from kidney disease to varicose veins, to following a high-protein low-carbohydrate diet.

DETOX DIETS

Looking at many current detox diets, we believe they are likely to result in deficiency conditions whereby the intake of certain vitamins, minerals and other essential nutrients such as omega-3 fatty acids is too low for good health. This is particularly likely if the diets are used for too long. Moreover, many detox diets fail to consider how food is grown, produced, prepared, treated and manufactured, and the man-made chemicals that become incorporated during such processes.

STARVATION DIETS

These are extreme variants of the detox diets and can have even more serious effects on the body than detox diets.

CRASH AND EXTREME DIETS

Repeated crash dieting is also unhealthy and can increase the risk of heart disease. Moreover, the quick weight loss achieved initially tends to be short lived, and is often accompanied by increased cholesterol levels. The problem is that when we eat less food our metabolic rate, which controls the rate at which we burn off calories, falls.

ANTI-CANCER DIETS

These diets may make one or more of the following recommendations – which show a poor understanding of science.

1 Giving up fruit on the basis that it contains sugar.

This is nonsense, but stems from the fact that cancer cells are very inefficient in making energy compared to normal healthy cells, so they use far more glucose. Proponents of such diets argue that starving cancer cells of fruit starves them of sugar and hence glucose. All carbohydrates produce glucose when they are metabolised however – indeed the brain uses glucose as its principal fuel and would rapidly shut down without it. While we recommend strongly that no one, and certainly not cancer patients, should eat refined white carbohydrates (such as white sugar, flour or bread), unrefined sugar, molasses and fresh fruit are actually very good for health. Moreover, in addition to powerful antioxidants, fruit contains lots of chemicals that fight cancer. For example, pineapple contains the powerful protein-digesting enzyme bromelain, which has been shown to reduce tumours and inhibit metastasis by blocking a protein that cancer cells need, as well as by activating specific anti-cancer immune cells. Papaya contains a similar enzyme called papayain. Recent research has also shown that natural antifungal substances known as salvestrols that are present in high quantities in organically produced fruit interact with an enzyme known as CYP1B1 that is present in all precancerous and cancer cells, but does not occur in healthy cells. The combination of salvestrols with CYP1B1 produces a chemical that helps to convert cancer cells into normal cells.

2 Giving up aubergines (eggplants), potatoes, tomatoes and chilli peppers on the basis that they belong to the deadly nightshade (*Solanaceae*) family.

The chemical lycopene, which is present in red vegetables, especially tomatoes, is a powerful anti-cancer chemical and populations that consume large quantities of these vegetables, such as in the Mediterranean region, generally have much lower rates of cancer. The capsaicin chemicals in chilli peppers have also been shown to have powerful anti-cancer properties, including against leukaemia. The only possible link known between these vegetables and cancer is from eating fried potatoes such as chips or crisps, because a carcinogen known as acrylamide can form during the cooking process.

3 Giving up all wheat.

While the gliadin storage proteins in wheat may cause symptoms in people with coeliac disease there are no known links between organically produced wholegrain wheat and cancer. Indeed, wheat contains a wide range of phytochemicals concentrated in the bran and germ that reduce cancer risk. Problems arise if wheat is refined, however, because the concentration of anti-cancer chemicals is reduced by 200 to 300 times in the process. Moreover, consuming highly processed bread and cereals floods the body with sugar and stimulates it to increase levels of the growth factor IGF-1, which is strongly linked to increased risk for many types of cancer.

4 Giving up soya on the basis that it contains phyto-oestrogens – advice that is often accompanied by a recommendation to consume dairy products such as yoghurt (now often called probiotics) instead.

Yoghurt was one of the first substances to be linked to ovarian cancer by doctors at Harvard University, and many laboratory experiments indicate that casein (cow's milk protein) promotes cancer cells, whereas soya does not. Animal milk generally contains cancer-promoting growth factors and animal steroid hormones such as oestrogen, while soya, like other beans and peas and fruit and vegetables, contains phyto-oestrogens described by the authoritative Royal Society as protective against cancer. Populations consuming diets high in soya or other beans and peas generally have lower rates of all hormone-dependent cancers.

5 Taking lots of man-made vitamin and mineral pills (often marketed under their own name and/or sold at great profit).

All the scientific evidence indicates a worse outcome for cancer sufferers taking such supplements.

A non-evidence-based approach

Any doctor or therapist making the recommendations described above is failing to use an evidence-based approach based on the mainstream peer-reviewed scientific literature and you should be extremely cautious about following such advice.

BACKGROUND TO THE PLANT PROGRAMME – THE CHINESE WAY

The Plant Programme diet in *Eating for Better Health*, like the previous Plant Programme devised specifically to prevent and treat breast and prostate cancer, is based on a modified Chinese diet. The Chinese diet has been shown to be one of the healthiest in the world. Like Chinese medicine, it has evolved over thousands of years of observation, practical experience and continued refinement, and the knowledge has been handed down from generation to generation.

The traditional Chinese diet provides an excellent response to nutritional and environmental problems and has sustained the Chinese population for thousands of years so that they have become the most biologically successful people on Earth. They have traditionally used organic methods of farming, by separating their waste streams so that any animal or human waste is recycled back into agricultural land, minimising contamination and the need for fertiliser.

Our diet is based on this well-tried, traditional, observation-based diet of China and other parts of southeast Asia, where rates of chronic diseases have traditionally been very low (though, as in many developing countries, chronic diseases are increasing there along with Westernisation).

PRINCIPLES OF THE TRADITIONAL CHINESE DIET

Until recent years, when Westernisation began to take hold in China and southeast Asia, their diet was characterised by:

- A high calorie intake. The Chinese consumed more calories than the Americans (though they were much less obese).
- A low fat intake. Only 14 per cent of calories in the average Chinese diet came from fat, compared with almost 36 per cent in the West, and much of the fat in the Chinese diet was 'good fat' from vegetables or fish rather than unhealthy saturated fats from meat or dairy products.
- A very high ratio of vegetable protein to animal protein, about 10:1, which compares with a ratio of 1:2 or lower in the USA and Europe. Animal protein made up about 11 per cent of the

average American diet but only 1 per cent of the average Chinese diet (and most of that was from fish, eggs, chicken, duck or pork, rather than beef or dairy). Vegetables such as soya beans were traditionally the main source of protein in China and much of southeast Asia.

- A high fibre intake, reflecting the large amount of vegetable foods in the diet. The Chinese consumed an average 34g of fibre a day (with no evidence of iron or other mineral deficiency), compared with the average fibre intake of Americans of only 10–12g a day. Remember, all unrefined plant food contains fibre, while no animal food contains any fibre. It has been known since the 1950s and was confirmed recently by the European Prospective Investigation of Cancer (EPIC) that a high-fibre, plant-based diet dramatically reduces the risk of colorectal cancer.

- A complete lack of dairy produce of any sort. Recent studies in the UK have shown that about 80 per cent of the dietary intake of female steroid hormones such as oestrogen and progesterone is from dairy produce, the remainder coming from other animal produce in the diet. Cow's milk has been shown to contain over thirty-five different hormones and eleven growth factors, many of which are directly implicated in human reproductive and other types of cancer. Growth factors for laboratory research are normally obtained from milk or cheese whey. Milk also concentrates hormone-mimicking pollutants from the environment, which could directly or indirectly damage health. The content of calcium in cow's milk is approximately five times that in human milk, and this causes a range of health problems.

- A high content of vitamins, minerals, omega-3 fatty acids, plant chemicals (phytochemicals) and other healthy nutrients, which are protective against a wide range of diseases.

- A high content of freshly picked vegetables and freshly killed animals and fish. If you have eaten in a restaurant in China you will know that if you order fish, it is taken out of a fish tank and killed for your meal.

- An alcohol intake that makes up 5 per cent of total calories. This is similar to that of the USA, where it makes up approximately 7 per cent of total calories.

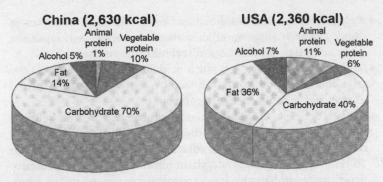

Figure 1 Comparison of oriental and US diets in the mid-1980s

In Japan, where the traditional diet was fairly similar to that of China, they consider that a healthy diet is based on eating at least thirty different ingredients a day. This contrasts with the diet of the average American, for whom 40 per cent of their diet is from dairy. Anyone who has visited the USA and watched television there will recall being bombarded with advertisements for treatments for everything from stomach acidity to headaches, as well as joint problems and many other illnesses – suggesting that their diet is not a healthy one.

Our diet is based on proportions of animal and vegetable protein, fat and carbohydrate similar to those of the traditional Chinese diet. It also follows the principles of the Japanese diet by including a good variety of ingredients, which ensures an intake of a wide range of essential nutrients and also minimises repeated exposure to any particular harmful chemical.

We shall first describe the basic principles of our diet, set out as ten food factors, before describing various disease conditions. We show how the basic dietary principles are customised to each disease condition.

It is perhaps worth emphasising here that chronic diseases such as Alzheimer's, as well as autoimmune conditions such as multiple sclerosis, cardiovascular disease, hormone-dependent (breast, ovarian, prostate and testicular) cancer, diverticulitis and many other diseases follow the Western diet geographically and in time. Such diseases show associations with:

- Pesticide spray and residues, and other chemical additives in food; research suggests links with Alzheimer's, parkinsonism, chronic fatigue syndrome and several types of cancer.
- A diet that generates too much acid in the body and too little alkalinity – a risk factor for many diseases, including mental illness and musculoskeletal problems.
- A diet deficient in soluble and insoluble fibre. Fibre helps to protect against digestive-tract diseases including colorectal cancer and lowers cholesterol levels. All unrefined plant products contain fibre; no animal products contain fibre. A diet with insufficient fruit and vegetables also lacks the antioxidants and phytochemicals that help to prevent cancer and cardiovascular disease.
- A diet too high in refined carbohydrates – a risk factor for high blood sugar, obesity and type-2 diabetes, and hence for heart and eye diseases including blindness.
- A diet too high in animal protein, which can generate damaging homocysteine – a risk factor for Alzheimer's, stroke and heart attacks. Such A diet also makes the body too acid.
- A diet too high in saturated and trans-fats and too low in essential fatty acids, especially omega-3 fatty acids. Such a diet is a risk factor for cancer, heart disease, multiple sclerosis and mental illness.
- A diet too high in salt, which is linked to high blood pressure and cardiovascular disease.
- A diet too low in healthy fresh herbs and spices such as basil, parsley, ginger and garlic, which are full of powerful anti-oxidants, minerals and beneficial phytochemicals that protect against many physical and mental diseases.
- A diet with too much refined white sugar, which is linked to type-2 diabetes, or too many artificial sweeteners, which are linked to some types of cancer and anxiety states.
- A diet that provides too much calcium, which is a risk factor for Alzheimer's and parkinsonism, or is deficient in magnesium, other essential trace elements such as iodine, lithium and selenium, or vitamins, including the B vitamins – a risk factor for heart disease, chronic fatigue syndrome and mental illness.
- A diet with too many fizzy drinks, or too much alcohol or caffeine, which is linked to a range of physical and mental illnesses.

TAKING CONTROL OF YOUR HEALTH – THE FOOD FACTORS

Here are ten simple but science-based food factors to help you prevent and treat illness.

- Food Factor 1 – Organic foods and man-made chemicals
- Food Factor 2 – Balancing your diet
- Food Factor 3 – Vegetables and fruit
- Food Factor 4 – Healthy sources of carbohydrates
- Food Factor 5 – Healthy sources of protein
- Food Factor 6 – Healthy sources of fats
- Food Factor 7 – Healthy seasonings
- Food Factor 8 – Healthy sweeteners
- Food Factor 9 – Supplements
- Food Factor 10 – Healthy drinks

FOOD FACTOR 1 – ORGANIC FOODS AND MAN-MADE CHEMICALS

Sometimes people who advocate organic food are dismissed as middle-class food fanatics, with no rational or scientific basis for their concerns. We would like to tell you why this caricature is wrong and why it is important that you insist on as much high-quality organic food as possible. Organic food costs a bit more, but for the sake of your health it is worth the extra expense.

Organic, or biological, agriculture is a system of food production designed to minimise the use of agrochemical inputs and avoid damage to the environment and wildlife. The emphasis is on the life cycle of the total environment, and organic food is generally fresh, living food. The use of chemical additives is also severely restricted or banned in the manufacture of organic food, whereas in most processed foods, the content of fibre, vitamins, minerals, natural colours or other natural constituents has been removed or significantly damaged and replaced with man-made chemicals.

Conventional agriculture relies on the input of large amounts of agrochemicals, and food production and manufacture can involve a great deal of processing and refining and the further use of chemical additives. Such food is often designed to have a long shelf life: 'fossil food'.

Pesticides used in conventional agriculture can inhibit the activity of chemicals responsible for important processes in the body (organophosphates derived from nerve gas, for example, inhibit an important neurotransmitter) or they may work by sending the wrong signals to the nervous system. Some, such as Paraquat, may increase free-radical production in the body, while others work by disturbing the pH gradient across cell membranes. Others may dissolve in the cell membranes or disturb their ionic balance. Strong acids, strong alkalis, bromine (bromine compounds are often used to fumigate soils before planting strawberries) and chlorine gas are toxic because they dissolve and destroy tissue. Moreover, many man-made chemicals, including some pesticides, are now known to have endocrine-disrupting properties, which means that they interfere with the functioning of the sex-steroid hormones, oestrogen or testosterone, or with thyroid function.

Most of the pesticides used now are systemic; that is they are distributed throughout the plant and will not wash off. If you eat such foods you cannot avoid pesticide residues building up in your body, although new research shows that these residues decline markedly within six weeks in those switching to organically produced food. Genetically modified (GM) foods such as American corn generally contain even more pesticides, including the systemic nicotinyls (neonicotinoids) suspected by many scientists of devastating the honey bee population. The seed for GM crops is generally so expensive now that farmers do not want to risk crop failure so they spray systemic pesticides on such crops every few days.

In addition to the plethora of chemicals now used in conventional arable farming, farmed animals are frequently treated with antibiotics, sometimes for growth promotion rather than disease control, and with anti-parasitic substances. Organic farming and production ban or regulate the use of all such chemicals.

Let us use farmed fish as an example of some differences between organically produced and conventionally produced food. Organic production bans the use of artificial pigments, which are used to make salmon pink and which can damage the human eye (organic producers use shrimp shell instead). The Soil Association also bans growth regulators, appetite stimulants and other veterinary medicines including hormones, whereas some conventionally farmed fish such as trout are routinely treated with female sex hormones to improve their taste. The use of copper-based and other poisonous materials to paint cages is also banned in organic fish farming, as is the use of synthetic pesticides and avermectin products. The latter, which are used to control sea lice and other parasites in farmed fish, are fat-soluble, cross the blood-brain barrier and interfere with the activity of one of the brain's main neurotransmitters, GABA (nicknamed the 'tranquillity neurotransmitter'). In organic fish farming, the aim is to control parasites mainly by using salt baths.

Recent work at Newcastle University's food centre suggests there is an increased level of nutritionally beneficial substances, including vitamins and antioxidants, in organically produced food. Substances that increase the plant's protection to insects are also increased, thereby reducing the need for pesticides. These include anti-cancer chemicals such as the salvestrols, levels of which are much higher in organically produced fruit.

Guidelines

- Eat food that is produced and prepared organically to the standards of a reputable organisation, such as the Soil Association, to reduce your intake of man-made chemicals, especially pesticides ('cide' is from the Latin meaning 'to kill'). The Soil Association's symbol is a circle with the words SOIL ASSOCIATION around the top and ORGANIC STANDARD round the bottom, and a sort of curly, triangular design inside the circle.
  - ○ It is possible to buy a wide range of organic fruit and vegetables in most areas of the UK. If necessary, use the Internet to find a local supplier.
  - ○ Grain products, including rice, are often heavily sprayed, so they can contain pesticide residues, and processed food made with maize can contain organophosphate residues.
  - ○ In the USA, strawberries have been called the most pesticide-ridden food.
  - ○ Banana growing frequently involves the use of pesticides that are implicated in birth defects or are neurotoxins.
  - ○ Pesticide Action Network (PAN) UK lists the UK's ten worst foods for residues on its website www.pan-uk.org as: flour, potatoes, bread, apples, pears, grapes, strawberries, green

beans, tomatoes and cucumber. Their advice is to keep eating at least five servings of fruit and vegetable a day; consider replacing the items on their top-ten list with organic produce; increase your consumption of fruit and vegetables least likely to contain pesticide residues; make your concerns known to your local supermarket; grow your own fruit and vegetables (many people have a garden, an allotment or even a balcony, where they can grow some vegetables in a growbag).

- Do not consume even organically produced dairy, because it will still contain growth factors and hormones.
- Eat only organically produced meat, especially in the case of fat meats such as pork and duck, and even with organic produce discard the fat and skin before cooking because this is where most environmental pollutants accumulate.
- Avoid all dairy produce, certain fish-liver oils and conventionally farmed fish, especially carnivorous fish such as salmon (newly published research shows that farmed salmon contains high levels of polychlorinated biphenyls (PCBs) – which can produce adverse health effects, including liver damage, skin irritations, reproductive and development effects and cancer – and detectable levels of contaminants, such as brominated flame retardants, and the pesticides DDT and hexachlorocyclohexane). It is easy to recognise wild or organically produced salmon, because the flesh is much paler than the luminously orange pink of chemically fed fish.
- Cut out or cut down on manufactured convenience food, especially anything with E numbers in it.
- Use brown unrefined cereal products, including flour and products made from it such as bread, cakes and pasta.
- Ensure that everything is as fresh, natural and unaltered as possible to avoid the need for vitamin or mineral supplements.
- Eat freshly prepared food.
- Avoid food that has been overprocessed, including overcooking in the home using excessive boiling, stewing or baking. Do not use a pressure cooker or microwave oven.
- Avoid tinned food and pre-prepared convenience meals. Frozen foods are usually OK, and there is an increasing range of organically produced food available in bottles, jars and tins, which are fine occasionally.

• Do not use plastic, especially soft plastic wrappings, or eat food from tins with plastic linings. Minimise your intake of food from tins generally. Phthalates used in plastics and bisphenol A from the plastic lining of tin cans are oestrogenic, with implications for female reproductive cancer and the health of baby boys. They are also implicated in depression and anxiety. Most of the results of tests that Jane has carried out on the urine samples of her patients show high to exceptionally high levels of phthalates.

Research at Southampton University has once again confirmed a link between food additives and hyperactivity in children, so it would seem sensible for adults to avoid these too – especially if you suffer from anxiety or mood swings. The ones particularly implicated are described in the table on pages 24–25.

Other uses of some of the azo dyes used for food colouring include soap, moisturisers, cosmetics, shampoos, crayons and stamp dyes. Beware! Both prescription and over-the-counter drugs and remedies such as cough mixtures can have these colorants – sometimes a whole cocktail of them. They may be combined with aspartame, which can produce unpleasant symptoms in some people (see page 43). Many people attribute low mood or agitation to illness when it is really due to the pills they are popping. Try to use some of the natural remedies described in this book.

> Organically produced food keeps its natural colour, or is coloured by natural colorants such as beetroot juice or betacarotene.

FOOD FACTOR 2 – BALANCING YOUR DIET

There are two kinds of balance to keep in mind. First, the balance of animal and vegetable protein, animal and vegetable carbo-hydrate, and animal and vegetable fat, where we recommend similar proportions to those of the traditional Chinese diet, and, secondly, the balance of acid-generating to alkali-generating foods. One of the biggest problems with the Western diet is that it contains far too much protein – especially animal protein. It is

Table 1 Food additives

	Description	Uses	May be found in	Known and suspected health effects, in addition to hyperactivity	Other comments
Sunset yellow (E110)	Synthetic coal tar and orange/ yellow azo dye	Colouring	Orange squash and other soft drinks, orange jelly, marzipan, Swiss roll, apricot jam, marmalade, lemon curd, sweets, packet soups, trifle mix, breadcrumbs, cheese sauce mix, yoghurts, as well as some over-the-counter medications, including pain killers. It is used together with Amaranth (E123) to produce a brown colour for hot chocolate mixes, chocolates and caramel	Allergic reactions with symptoms of gastric upset, diarrhoea, nausea and vomiting, nettle rash and swelling of the skin	Banned in Norway and Finland; to be phased out in UK
Carmoisine (E122)	Synthetic red azo dye	Colouring	Blancmange, jellies, marzipan, Swiss rolls, jams and preservatives, sweets, brown sauce, yoghurts, soups, breadcrumbs, cheesecake mixes and some mouthwashes	Allergic and intolerance reactions, with gastric upsets, nausea and diarrhoea; nettle rash and water retention	Commonly used in the UK but to be phased out; banned in Japan, Norway, Sweden and the USA
Tartrazine (E102)	Synthetic lemon yellow azo dye, very commonly used because it is inexpensive	Colouring	Confectionery/candy, soft drinks (including fruit squashes and cordials), crisps, biscuits, products with glycerine and honey, instant puddings, snack biscuits, cereals (including cornflakes and muesli), soup cubes and mixes, some rice brands, ice cream, pops, lollies, chewing gum, marzipan, jam, jelly, marmalade, mustard, horseradish sauce, yoghurt, noodles, pickles, Chinese food (including egg noodles), vitamin capsules and tablets, antacids, medical capsules and some prescription drugs	Allergic and intolerance reactions, such as asthma attacks and hives; by ingestion or skin contact, especially in asthmatics and those sensitive to aspirin; anxiety, clinical depression, migraine, blurred vision, sleep disturbance and general weakness	One study in Australia has linked 'artrazine to obsessive compulsive disorder; it is also used with Brilliant Blue (E133) or Green S to produce various green shades, which may be found in tinned vegetables such as mushy peas

Ponceau (E124)	Red azo dye	Colouring	Used in a range of processed and convenience foods; found in Chinese manufactured sweets and confectionery; intensifies asthma by releasing histamine; causes intolerance symptoms, especially in those allergic to aspirin	It is considered carcinogenic in the USA, Finland and Norway	
Quinoline yellow (E104)	Yellow food dye	Colouring	Ice creams, lollies, cough sweets, scotch eggs, smoked haddock; also used as tattoo pigment	Contact dermatitis	Banned in Japan and USA; to be phased out in UK
Allura Red AC (E129)	Red azo food dye, derived from coal tar	Colouring	Alcoholic beverages, fish products, soft drinks, confectionery, medications (including for children); also used as tattoo pigment	Can cause nettle rash, nausea, breathing difficulties and even anaphylactic shock	The non-food grade product can contain a carcinogen banned in Denmark, Belgium, France, Germany, Switzerland, Sweden and Austria; to be phased out in UK
Sodium benzoate (E211)	Preservative	Bacterio-static and fungistatic in acid conditions	Used to preserve salad dressings containing vinegar, fizzy drinks, jams, preserves, fruit juices, pickles, condiments and some cough syrups and pet foods; also used in fireworks, silver polish and some mouth washes	Decreased intelligence in children; nettle rash (urticaria); in combination with vitamin C (E300) may release benzene (a potent carcinogen); may damage DNA (including in cell mitochondria), which causes cell death: many diseases including parkinsonism and other neurodegenerative disorders have been linked to such a process	

worth remembering that the main use of protein is to repair worn-out cells and tissues, and to provide messenger molecules such as growth factors (which control cell growth, development and repair) and neurotransmitters (which enable the neurons in the brain to communicate with each other). According to the eminent nutritional scientist Professor T. Colin Campbell, the intake of protein in the diet should be about 10–11 per cent. The traditional Chinese diet contains an ideal 11 per cent protein, including about 1 per cent animal protein. By way of contrast, we may note that many people in the West consume up to 16 per cent of their calories as protein, and some eat an unhealthy 20 per cent or more if they follow a low carbohydrate fad diet. (There is more about healthy sources of protein in Food Factor 5 below.) Most of our daily food intake, i.e. some 70–75 per cent of total calorie intake, should be complex, unrefined carbohydrates. These are the real fuel foods that supply the energy for the brain and muscles (see further under Food Factor 4 below). We also need some fats – about 15 per cent of total calories – to maintain the optimum structure and function of the brain and nerves, cell walls and some messenger molecules. Fats can also be used to generate energy and to keep us warm. The right fats can act as highly effective electrical and thermal insulators in our bodies, but the wrong ones clog up our arteries and cause the nervous system to malfunction (see further under Food Factor 6 below).

The acid–alkali balance in the body is crucial to our physical and mental health. One of the advantages of the traditional Chinese diet is that it will not cause acid to accumulate in the body, which can lead to many disease conditions. The latest research suggests that maintaining the balance between acid-generating and alkali-generating food is crucial for health and helps to protect against many chronic diseases, ranging from bone disorders such as osteoporosis, kidney stones and urinary-tract infections, to anxiety and depression. The aim is to try to achieve a balance between acid-generating and alkali-generating food intake (see below for some guidelines) to keep the blood just to the alkaline side of neutral. This is a top priority for the body, because if the blood becomes too acid or alkaline we become ill; the range of pH that can be tolerated is very small.

There is much information on how to balance the pH of the body using food in the alternative medical literature, but this is generally not based on sound science. Recently, however, a leading German institute, the Institute of Clinical Nutrition in Dortmund, concerned with research into clinical nutrition has for the first time developed authoritative, scientifically based information on which foods generate acidity or alkalinity in the human body. The chart on pages 28–28 is based on their findings.

> For the first time, we have a truly scientific method for determining the acidity or alkalinity that foods generate in our bodies, so that we can balance our diets effectively.

The chart based on the new German research overturns previous poorly based alternative medical information on which foods are acid- or alkali-generating. Much of the old alternative literature referred to 'acid-ash' and 'alkali-ash' foods, reflecting the totally unsatisfactory method of burning the food and shaking it in distilled water before determining its pH. Some of the key differences between the new scientific result and the old classification are that:

- Many dairy foods, previously considered as alkali-generating, are shown to be acid-generating foods, especially hard cheese which is the most acid-generating food identified. Hard cheese generally is up to three times more acid-generating than beef, for example, and almost all dairy produce is moderately to very strongly acid-producing. Whey is the only exception, but this should not be consumed because it contains biochemically active substances such as growth factors, which are implicated in breast cancer and prostate cancer.
- Other acid- and strongly acid-generating foods include meat and meat products, fish, eggs, especially their yolks, and other protein foods including some cereals and soya products.
- Bread, white rice and pulses such as peas and lentils are moderately acid forming, although whole wheat is shown to be much less acid-producing than previously thought.
- Most fats and oils are close to neutral.

(Continued on page 30)

Table 2 Potential renal acid load (PRAL) of foods and beverages (related to 100g portions)*

	Very strongly alkaline	−20 Strongly alkaline	−10 Alkaline	−5 Moderately alkaline	−0.5 Nearly neutral	0.5 Moderately acid	5 Acid	10 Strongly acid	20 Very strongly acid
Herbs and spices	Parsley, dried −62.4 Basil, dried −57.9 Ginger −23	Curry powder −19.9 Black pepper −19.7		Chives −3.6					
Fruits and juices	Raisins −21		Blackcurrants −6.5 Bananas −5.5	Apricots −4.8 Kiwi fruit −4.1 Tomato juice −3.8 Cherries −3.6 Orange juice −2.9 Pears −2.9 Oranges −2.7 Pineapple −2.7 Lemon juice −2.5 Peaches −2.4 Apple juice −2.2 Apples −2.2 Strawberries −2.2 Watermelon −1.9					
Vegetables		Spinach −14	Celery −5.2	Carrots, young −4.9 Zucchini −4.6 Cauliflower −4.0 Potatoes, old −4.0 Radish, red −3.7 Eggplant −3.4 Tomatoes −3.1 Beans, green −3.1 Lettuce −2.5 Chicory −2.0 Leeks −1.8 Lettuce, iceberg −1.6 Onions −1.5 Mushrooms −1.4 Peppers −1.4 Broccoli −1.2 Cucumber −0.8	Asparagus −0.4				
Beverages				Red wine −2.4 Mineral water (example) −1.8 Coffee −1.4 White wine, dry −1.2 Grape juice −1	Cocoa −0.4 Tea −0.3 Beer, draught −0.2 Beer, stout −0.1 Mineral water (example) −0.1 Cola 0.4	Beer, pale 0.9			

Fats and oils			Margarine −0.5 Olive oil 0.0 Sunflower-seed oil 0.0				
Sugars, sweets and preserves		Marmalade −1.5	Honey −0.3 Sugar, white −0.1	Chocolate, milk 2.4 Madeira cake 3.7			
Legumes and nuts	Soya flour −5.9	Soya beans −4.7 Natto −3.2 Hazelnuts −2.8	Soya milk −0.3 Soya bean, sprouted raw 0.3	Peas 1.2 Mori-Nu tofu 2.0 Tofu 3.4 Lentils 3.5 Soya sauce 4.5	Miso 6.9 Tempeh 8.2 Tofu, prepared with calcium sulphate 8.3 Walnuts 6.8 Peanuts, plain 8.3		
Grain products				Rice, white, boiled 1.7 Bread, wheat wholemeal 1.8 Crispbread, rye 3.3 Bread, wheat, white 3.7 Bread, wheat, mixed 3.8 Bread, rye, mixed 4.0 Bread, rye 4.1 Rice, white 4.6	Rye flour, whole 5.9 Cornflakes 6.0 Noodles, egg 6.4 Spaghetti, white 6.5 Wheat flour, white 6.9 Spaghetti, wholemeal 7.3 Wheat flour, wholemeal 8.2	Oat flakes 10.7 Rice, brown 12.5	
Meat					Frankfurters 6.7 Beef, lean 7.8 Pork, lean 7.9 Chicken, meat 8.7 Steak, lean and fat 8.8 Veal 9.0 Turkey, meat 9.9	Luncheon meat 10.2 Liver sausage 10.6 Salami 11.6 Corned beef 13.2	
Fish and eggs				Eggwhites 1.1	Haddock 6.8 Herring 7.0 Cod 7.1 Eggs, whole 8.2	Trout 10.8	Eggyolks 23.4
Dairy products				Butter 0.6 Ice cream 0.6 Milk, whole 0.7 Milk, evaporated 1.1 Creams, fresh, sour 1.2 Yoghurt, fruit 1.2 Yoghurt, plain 1.5 Soft cheese 4.3	Cottage cheese 8.7	Fresh cheese 11.1 Camembert 14.6 Cheese, Gouda 18.6 Hard cheese 19.2	Cheese, cheddar-type, reduced fat 26.4 Processed cheese 28.7 Parmesan 34.2

PRAL values are expressed in milli-equivalents of X per 100g portion of food consumed, where X is the percentage of principal acids (chloride (Cl) + phosphate (PO_4) + sulphate (SO_4)) minus the percentage of principal bases (sodium (Na) + potassium (K) + calcium (Ca) + magnesium (Mg)) present in the food.
*Remer, T. and Manz, F., 1995. Potential renal acid load of foods and its influence on urine pH. J Am Diet Assoc, 95, 791–797; and Remer, personal communication.

- Almost all fruit and vegetables, even tomatoes and citrus fruits (including lemons), which alternative practitioners have always classified as acid-generating, are alkali-generating when metabolised the body. Dried fruits such as raisins are particularly alkali-generating unless they are preserved in sulphur compounds.
- Spices such as ginger and garlic, and dried herbs such as parsley and coriander, are very alkali-generating.
- Beverages low in phosphorus, such as spirits, red and white wine and beer, are neutral to slightly alkali-generating, so that moderate alcohol intake is unlikely to damage the overall balance of the diet. Tea, including herbal teas such as peppermint, many mineral waters and soya milk are all moderately alkali-generating or nearly neutral, but fizzy drinks high in phosphorus are acid-producing.

The most acid-producing, and therefore most bone-damaging, foods consumed in the Western diet include hard and processed cheeses, egg yolk (so be careful with the egg mayonnaise!) and, to a lesser extent, tinned and processed meats. The most protective foods, because of their alkali production in the body, are fruit and vegetables, herbs and spices.

Guidelines

Five things to bear in mind are:

- The ideal ratio for maintaining optimum health is 60:40 alkali-generating to acid-generating food intake. Research in North America suggests that the average American eats a diet where this ratio is an amazing 15:85 in favour of acid-generating foods. Such an acid-generating diet creates thicker, more viscous blood and lymphatic congestion, and in the long term will damage bone and tissue.
- Many herbs and spices have been used for a long time in Eastern cooking and help to neutralise the acid generated by meat, fish and cereals such as rice.
- Diets such as the traditional Chinese one, which is based mainly on vegetable rather than animal protein (see Figure 1), are far less acid-generating than typical Western diets, and are easier to

balance – just imagine how much spinach you would need to eat to balance a portion of hard cheese.

- It is essential to have some acid-forming foods in the diet, or your protein intake may be too low and other conditions, caused by excessive alkalinity, can be caused.
- Every human being is unique. We do not all metabolise food in exactly the same way. Depending on our ancestry and our genes, we may have different nutritional requirements. So you should use Table 2 as a guide to find the dietary regime that is right for you.

Overall, the message is to keep the consumption of animal protein low relative to that of vegetable protein. Good sources of vegetable protein are discussed under Food Factor 5. While you don't need to balance every individual meal, selecting which foods to eat together can reduce gas, indigestion and bloating. If you have this problem, don't drink with your meals and always eat fruit separately: leave at least half an hour after a meal before you drink anything or eat fruit. Combining cereals with meat can also cause problems. Eating fish or meat with vegetables should be fine, as should a totally vegan meal, such as pulses, grains, tortillas or a cheese-free pizza with tomato sauce and vegetables. Eating a salad with most foods is fine.

FOOD FACTOR 3 – VEGETABLES AND FRUIT

For a long time it has been recognised that diets high in vegetables, fruit, seeds and nuts reduce the risk of cancer, cardiovascular disease and diabetes. Some of these effects are attributed to phytochemicals (i.e. plant chemicals) designed to protect the plant against insects. Raw vegetables and fruit, sprouted grains and other types of seeds all contain enzymes that are important nutrients and help the body's metabolism. These living foods are the antithesis of 'fossil food'. A recent survey of more than 30,000 people carried out by Optimum Nutrition UK found that fresh vegetable and fruit consumption was positively correlated with all indicators of good health. They recommend consuming at least eight to ten servings of fresh fruit and vegetables a day. They also recommend three portions of fresh, raw seeds and nuts a day. The UK Government recommendation of five portions of fruit and vegetables a day, which includes prepared fruit and vegetables, is therefore wholly inadequate for healthy living.

Vegetables and fruit contain a powerhouse of minerals, vitamins, antioxidants, enzymes and phytochemicals. Most fruits are 85–90 per cent water, which is good for cleansing, and they are naturally low in calories and fat and contain soluble fibre, which helps to lower blood cholesterol levels and regulate blood sugar. A diet high in fruit and vegetables aids detoxification and lowers blood fats. The high fibre content also helps bowel movement and proper functioning of the immune system. Many act as 'prebiotics', which the latest research shows are much more likely to encourage friendly bacteria to flourish in the gut and are much less risky than eating probiotics, especially dairy yoghurts.

Guidelines

- Eat as much fresh organic vegetable and fruit from as wide a range as possible.
- Eat red vegetables such as tomatoes, red peppers and chillies; and orange vegetables, including peppers, carrots, sweet potatoes and pumpkins. These are all high in carotenoids, which are powerful antioxidants.
- Eat lots of green vegetables, including spinach and cruciferous vegetables such as bok choy, cauliflower and broccoli.
- Eat vegetables as fresh and raw as possible and have at least eight to ten large portions of fruit and vegetables as salads or juices every day. One portion should be at least one piece of fresh fruit or a cup of raw vegetables.
- Eat a diet rich in phyto-oestrogens, including: soya and other beans and peas; whole-grain cereals, including flax and other seeds; nuts; berries such as cranberries; and sprouting seeds, especially alfalfa and bean sprouts. Because phyto-oestrogens lock on to receptors (in breast tissue, for example) but have only 0.02–0.001 per cent the activity of oestrogen, they are protective against cancer and osteoporosis and help with menopausal symptoms generally.
- Eat lots of garlic, onions and chives, which are alkaline, frequently rich in selenium and have many other health benefits.

- Fresh berries are especially good for health.
- Eat mushrooms, but try several varieties including shiitake, oyster and chestnut, rather than the usual commercial button mushrooms (see pages 62).
- Sea vegetables such as nori and wakame are especially good sources of vitamins and minerals, which Chinese sailors ate to prevent scurvy from at least the early fifteenth century.

Try to eat at least half your vegetables raw in salads or freshly made juices and the rest cook only lightly. An A to Z of the health benefits of some fruit and vegetables is given on page 48–71.

FOOD FACTOR 4 – HEALTHY SOURCES OF CARBOHYDRATES

Think of carbohydrates as your main source of energy. They are like the gas in your boiler or the petrol in your car. All carbohydrates are broken down in the body and reach individual cells as glucose. This is used in tiny organelles within cells called mitochondria, which behave like little boilers or engines to release energy as they 'burn' the glucose in a series of steps, finally producing carbon dioxide and water as waste products. If we use the wrong type of carbohydrates as fuel, we may fail to produce enough energy and the mitochondria may well start releasing toxic substances into our body that can damage our physical and mental wellbeing.

There are good carbohydrates – and carbohydrates that are bad for us. Healthy, or complex, carbohydrates contain naturally occurring starches that the body metabolises slowly as a source of energy. They are thought to help brain function and mood. Every human being needs whole unrefined complex carbohydrates in their diet. Good sources include: grains such as barley, buckwheat, brown rice, oats, maize, millet, quinoa, rye and wheat; potatoes, sweet potatoes and other starchy vegetables; and beans and other pulses (which are high in protein but contain almost no fat), nuts and seeds. All these foods are also rich in other nutrients and fibre. In contrast, sugary refined carbohydrates, such as white sugar, most commercial chocolate, cakes, biscuits, sweets and anything made with refined sugar or cereal flour consist mainly of empty calories and lack any other nutrients. In refining carbohydrates, any fluoride, which would protect the teeth, and chromium, which is needed for glucose-tolerance factor (thought to be protective against type-2 diabetes), are removed and added to animal feed.

Refined carbohydrates cause surges in blood glucose that can damage the pancreas, eventually leading to diabetes, and in the short term cause mood swings. Moreover, excessive amounts of these carbohydrates are stored as body fat and can lead to obesity. It has been suggested that such foods also stimulate the body to produce high levels of a growth factor called IGF-I, which is implicated in breast cancer and prostate cancer. Acne is suggested to be an indicator of the overproduction of IGF-I in the body. (Several people following our diet have reported that their acne has disappeared after giving up dairy produce and refined carbohydrates.) We wouldn't put the wrong fuel in the boiler or car, yet many people are prepared to put the wrong food into their body.

Most people in developing countries have traditionally relied on cereals as one of their main sources of foods, accompanied by low incidence of the diseases of affluence, including cancer and heart disease. Most diets aimed at disease prevention include plenty of whole-grain cereal foods such as bread and pasta. Clearly, if you are intolerant of or allergic to gluten you may need to avoid food and drink based on one or more of wheat, rye and barley, although many people can tolerate some gluten-containing foods better than others (wheat contains the most gluten). Good substitutes include rice and maize, and some new scientific evidence suggests that oats may be safe from a gluten viewpoint. Many nutritionists, especially alternative-health practitioners, recommend everyone against consuming wheat, partly because it is often linked to the establishment of settled farming – although barley, oats, maize and rice were also domesticated from wild cereal grasses at about the same time and have been used by farmers for thousands of years, albeit in an increasingly capital-intensive way. Perhaps wheat, which is now produced mainly by monocultural methods with a high input of chemicals and then greatly refined, is an example of how modern industrialised agriculture and food production can convert a good, nutrient-rich food into one that we are warned not to eat. In any case, it is a good idea to eat a range of whole-grain cereals rather than just wheat.

Whole grains contain a wide range of phytochemicals that reduce the risk of cancer. The active phytochemicals are concentrated in the bran and the germ, so that refining wheat causes a 200–300-fold loss in valuable phytochemical content. Tumour cells synthesise and accumulate cholesterol faster than normal cells, and some chemicals in whole-grain cereals (and fruit and vegetables) suppress tumour growth by limiting cholesterol synthesis. Other beneficial natural substances in whole grain induce the production of a detoxifying enzyme.

FOOD FACTOR 5 – HEALTHY SOURCES OF PROTEIN

Think of proteins as the building blocks, bricks, timber and glass of your house, or the bodywork and engine of your car. If you eat too much protein with too little carbohydrate, you are attacking the fabric of your body as it desperately tries to create energy from an unsuitable fuel.

Many protein molecules from animals are very large, made up from many amino acids sequenced following instructions from the DNA of the animal they came from. These should be broken down by the digestive system into the constituent amino acids, which are then reassembled according to instructions from our own DNA. The process has been likened to a process of breaking up a string of beads and reassembling them in a different order. Problems arise if our body has difficulty in breaking down proteins. The cow's milk protein casein (designed for an animal with five stomachs) can be difficult for humans to digest, especially if they do not have enough stomach acid (as a result of taking calcium tablets, for example). If fragments of a wrongly sequenced protein become incorporated in our tissues, problems can arise, especially with our immune system (see further under **Allergies** and **Autoimmune diseases**). Gluten, which is the main storage protein of wheat, also causes problems in some individuals.

After the Second World War there was an obsession with ensuring an adequate protein intake, and that meant school milk, and lots of meat, eggs and cheese, all strongly marketed on the basis of their high protein content. Interestingly, this type of high-protein diet has recently returned to favour to help weight loss.

Our parents considered a diet high in soya, other beans and pulses, cereal and nuts as comprising only second-class protein. All our findings, however, suggest that a diet with a high proportion of vegetable protein relative to animal protein is protective against many diseases including cancer and cardiovascular disease. For example, there is a dramatic decrease in the incidence of breast and prostate cancer and bone disease when the ratio of vegetable to animal protein in the diet is greater than 2:1.

One of the simplest and healthiest ways to help achieve this ratio is to substitute soya products for all dairy products. Be sure, however, to use only traditional soya food such as soya milk, tofu (bean curd), tempeh, natto or miso rather than soya that has been treated and flavoured with additives to resemble cheese or meat.

We recommend you try to keep to a maximum of one small portion of animal protein per day.

Guidelines

- Replace animal protein with vegetable protein from cereals and other seeds (such as alfalfa, pumpkin and sunflower seeds), pulses and nuts. Meals that combine cereals and pulses such as beans on toast or the Jamaican dish, rice and peas, provide the full range of proteins needed by the human body – but remember to eat some alkali-forming foods as well.
- Cut down on the amount of meat eaten – it should comprise less than 5 per cent of daily calorie intake for prevention and treatment of chronic illnesses and it should be from organically raised animals (try to keep to three small portions per week).
- Ensure that meat is cooked slowly and thoroughly. Meat that is raw inside contains hormones and growth factors, which would otherwise be broken down during cooking (while burning meat on the outside forms cancer-forming chemicals).
- Eat a little fish, especially oily fish, but make sure that it is wild or organically farmed. We recommend a maximum of one portion per week.
- Eat organic, free-range eggs in moderation.
- Eliminate all dairy produce, including the meat of dairy animals.

The humble soya bean

Despite recent alarmist information, mostly from unattributable websites, consuming soya as part of a well-balanced diet such as the Plant Programme is beneficial for most people.

In numerous scientific studies, soya beans have been shown to:

- protect cells from oxidative damage by free radicals, which can be a precursor to cancer and other chronic diseases;
- lower cholesterol without affecting levels of 'good' cholesterol, helping to prevent cardiovascular disease including stroke and coronary artery disease;
- reduce blood clotting, also helping to prevent heart attacks and strokes;
- reduce blood pressure (hypertension) by interfering with the production of some enzymes;
- regulate and stabilise oestrogen levels, thus helping to manage symptoms of menopause without the potentially dangerous side effects of HRT (the phyto-oestrogens in soya resemble human oestrogen but are significantly weaker so are considered protective against oestrogen-related cancer);
- inhibit and suppress the growth of several types of cancer cells and block enzymes that promote tumour growth;
- help to retain bone mass, thus guarding against osteoporosis, by reducing excretion of calcium – which also reduces the risk of kidney stones;
- boost the immune system;
- improve digestive function by helping the breakdown and absorption of fats, and by stimulating the growth of 'friendly' bacteria in the digestive tract;
- reduce the loss of protein in the urine in people suffering from kidney disorders.

Like many other familiar foods such as broccoli, Brussels sprouts, cabbage, cassava and turnip, soya contains 'goitrogens', which, if taken in excess, can affect thyroid function. Cooking helps to destroy these substances and an adequate intake of iodine from seafood such as fish or seaweed helps to prevent the problem. Rapeseed oil also contains goitrogens, but these are not neutralised by cooking or increasing iodine intake.

By doing this you will reduce your intake of hormones and growth factors from food that could promote cancer or cause overactive bone remodelling, for example. You will also reduce your exposure to unhealthy man-made chemicals and to pathogens such as salmonella and *E. coli*.

FOOD FACTOR 6 – HEALTHY SOURCES OF FATS

Fats, like proteins, should be considered as structural materials in the body. The brain comprises about 60 per cent fat, and the peripheral nervous system is also covered by a fatty substance called myelin, which protects nerves just as insulation like rubber or plastic protects electric cables. Other uses of fats are as energy storage (fats have 9 calories of energy per gram, compared with 4 calories per gram for carbohydrates and proteins), heat insulation and as a cushion for delicate organs such as the kidneys.

Many people are confused about the type and quantity of fats they should be eating and about the meaning of terms such as saturated and polyunsaturated. Fats are vital, but only in quantities and forms we would have consumed as hunter-gatherers. All fats are composed of fatty acids, some of which cannot be made in the body and therefore, like vitamins, must be obtained through the diet – these are the essential fatty acids. Fats are also necessary in the diet as a source of the fat-soluble vitamins, A, D, E and K. Fats are found in all body cells, in combination with other nutrients, and a healthy human brain and human breast comprise much fat. Excess fat stored in and around the heart, arteries and liver can be a problem, however.

There are four main types of dietary fat: monounsaturated and polyunsaturated fat – the good fats – and saturated fats and trans-fats – the bad fats. Some sources of these are shown in Table 3.

Among all the controversies about fats and oils, the message to minimise saturated fats in the diet has remained unchanged for decades. The Western diet now typically contains large quantities of trans-fatty acids (TFAs), which are somewhat similar in structure and behaviour to saturated fats. They originate primarily from hydrogenating oils, used to make margarines and spreads. Evidence suggests that they impair the metabolism of essential fatty acids.

Table 3 Dietary sources of fats

Saturated fats: eliminate** or reduce*	Trans-fatty acids (TFAs): eliminate or reduce	Monounsaturated fats: 'good fats'	Polyunsaturated fats: 'good fats'
Butter**	Margarine	Olives and olive oil	Vegetable oils
Cheese**	Cooking fats	Almonds	Sesame seeds
Milk**	Cakes	Pecan nuts	and oil
Red meats*	Highly processed	Peanuts	Safflower seeds
Fatty poultry such	foods, such as	Cashew nuts	and oil
as duck*	some commercial	Walnut	Sunflower seeds
Coconut oil*	mayonnaise,	Fish	and oil
Margarine**	dressings and		Corn oil
Palm oil*	creams		Wheat-germ oil
			Flax oil
			Pecan nuts
			Pine nuts
			Primrose oil
			Soya oil and beans
			Cold-water fish and
			fish-liver oils

Polyunsaturated and monounsaturated fats are generally liquid at room temperature. They should be bought cold-pressed and stored in dark bottles away from strong light, which causes them to become rancid and unhealthy. Monounsaturated oils such as olive oil are more stable and better for cooking. Polyunsaturated oils should never be heated to high temperature but can be added to stir-fries, for example, after cooking, while the dish is still warm, to add flavour.

The two classes of essential fatty acids (EFAs) that are polyunsaturated are the omega-6 (linoleic) and omega-3 (alpha linoleic) fatty acids.

There is growing evidence that omega-3 fatty acids help to reduce the risk of cardiovascular disease, including coronary heart disease, and help reduce blood triglyceride levels. The best sources include marine blue-green algae (this is where the fish obtain theirs from), mackerel and herring, and, to a lesser extent, salmon and trout (but ensure the latter two are wild or organically produced), and mussels. The essential omega-3 fatty acids are considered to help prevent and treat many disorders, including by:

- helping osteoarthritis and rheumatoid arthritis;
- controlling viral infections and improving immune function generally;
- reducing blood cholesterol and triglyceride levels;
- reducing blood clotting and lowering the risk of heart attack, stroke and hardening of the arteries;
- preventing abnormal heart rhythms;
- improving psoriasis (a distressing skin condition);
- improving immune response by lowering the harmful effects of body chemicals called prostaglandins, thus helping to prevent breast cancer and reduce the severity of migraine headaches;
- improving brain functioning, helping depression, anxiety and hyperactivity disorders;
- improving functioning of the glandular system.

Omega-6 fatty acids lower total blood cholesterol as well as levels of 'bad' LDL cholesterol. Most common vegetable oils, borage seed and evening primrose oil are high in omega-6 fatty acids.

Recent research is focusing less on absolute levels of omega-3 fatty acids and more on the ratio between them and omega-6 fatty acids. The latter tend to be high in Western diets, including in margarines and many processed foods.

All dark green leafy vegetables also contain omega-3 fatty acids, as do some plant-derived oils.

Table 4 Sources of essential fatty acids (amounts given in per cent)

Oils	Omega-3	Omega-6
Linseed (flax)	50–60	15–20
Walnut	5–10	20–30
Soya bean	5–10	40
Safflower	0.5	70
Sunflower	0.5	65
Corn	0.5	60
Cotton seed	0.5	50
Olive	0.5	10

Guidelines

- Keep total fat intake to less than 14 per cent of the daily calorie intake.

- Ensure you eat only good fats, because the types of fat consumed are very important.
- Saturated fat should be kept to an absolute minimum and replaced with mono- or polyunsaturated fats. This means eating more vegetables, nuts and fish and less red meat, dairy and eggs. Beef, for example, has a saturated to polyunsaturated ratio (S:P) of about 15:1; fish and poultry approximately 1:1; while vegetable fats in nuts and seeds have a ratio of S:P of less than 1:1.
- Polyunsaturated fats are excellent for salad dressings, for example, but they are relatively unstable and are damaged by light or cooking, when they can become oxidised and form damaging free radicals associated with increased risk of cancer and heart disease. The monounsaturated fats such as olive oil are better for cooking.
- Also avoid or minimise hydrogenated fats such as margarine and cooking oils, which can have increased saturated fat levels and unusable, unhealthy trans-fatty acids.

Eating out in restaurants or consuming fast foods may increase the total of unhealthy saturated-fat in the diet.

FOOD FACTOR 7 – HEALTHY SEASONINGS

Typically, the Western diet relies heavily on salt for seasoning. Processed and prepared food can contain particularly high levels of salt and other sodium-rich chemicals such as monosodium glutamate. High levels of salt and other sources of added sodium in the diet increase blood pressure and have long been linked to increased risk of cardiovascular disease.

Guidelines

- Read labels carefully and avoid all products that include salt, soda, sodium or the symbol Na on the label. The best-known source of sodium in the diet is salt, and in the UK, at least, there is pressure on the food industry to reduce levels in food. Other foods high in sodium include monosodium glutamate (MSG), a flavour enhancer with a meaty taste, baking soda, most types of tinned vegetables, many commercially prepared foods, diet soft drinks, foods with mould inhibitors, food with preservatives, meat tenderisers, saccharine, some medicines and toothpastes.

- Replace these unhealthy seasonings with lots of different fresh herbs. To take one example, basil, which is delicious with tomatoes for a summer salad, relieves a variety of digestive disorders including stomach cramps, vomiting and constipation, and should prevent intestinal parasites. (In very large amounts, however, it can cause anxiety and rapid heartbeat.) See pages 48–71 for more information on the health-giving properties of some herbs and spices.
- Eat spices, especially with meat, fish and egg dishes, since they help to counteract the acidity of such foods. Some spices contain anti-cancer chemicals, and many spices are good sources of trace minerals and contain useful amounts of chromium, copper, iron and other essential minerals.

FOOD FACTOR 8 – HEALTHY SWEETENERS

Some authors suggest that all sugars, from molasses to maple sugar and honey, should be avoided. While we recommend only moderate consumption (to help avoid obesity, diabetes and complications of these diseases), we consider the main problem relates to refined products, including processed honeys and white sugar. Professor Yudkin, a professor of human nutrition, famously termed the latter 'pure, white and deadly' in his 1972 book with that description as its title because it comprises mainly empty calories and has had essential trace nutrients such as vitamins and minerals (including chromium, which protects against diabetes, and fluoride, which, up to certain levels, protects against tooth decay) removed. Excess consumption of sugar can upset the body's mineral balance, suppress the immune system and cause anxiety and hyperactivity, and it is thought to be a key factor in the development of type-2 diabetes, heart disease, fatigue, obesity, depression and arthritis. It is also thought to be a factor in yeast infections.

Honey, where it has not been processed or heated, is a natural syrup comprising glucose, fructose and water with trace amounts of vitamins and minerals and other useful nutrients. It contains all its vitamins and minerals in natural proportions and is good for the immune system in those without blood-sugar problems. Heating kills enzymes, vitamins and other nutrients.

The herb, stevia, is one of the best natural sweeteners available. It is a concentrated natural sweetener derived from a South American shrub. It is not only completely safe but it also has healing properties. It has been used for centuries in South America and Asia and is the commonest calorie-free sweetener in Japan, where it is used in soft drinks, confectionery and cereals, for example. It should be the sweetener of choice for many types of illness, including diabetes.

Man-made sweeteners such as aspartame, which is manufactured using wood alcohol, and saccharine, which is manufactured from petroleum, have been suggested to cause a wide range of health problems.

Aspartame (E951) has been shown to form methanol in the body. Chronic low-level exposure to methanol has been linked to dizziness, ear-buzzing, nausea, upset digestion, vertigo, memory problems, numbness, insomnia, depression and pancreatitis. Moreover, some of the methanol can be converted to formaldehyde. Chronic formaldehyde exposure, even at low doses, has been shown to cause changes to the nervous system, poor immune function and DNA damage.

Guidelines

- Consume sugar only in moderation and ensure it is as unrefined as possible, bearing in mind that many brown sugars are simply dyed with caramel from burned white sugar.
- Avoid all substances that are products or by-products of sugar refining, such as white sugar (sucrose) and glucose.
- Avoid all artificial sweeteners such as aspartame, which is now one of the most widely used artificial sweeteners in the US and is widely used in diet drinks and many junk foods. Aspartame is marketed as Equal, NutraSweet and Canderel, and it is added to more than 5,000 foods and beverages worldwide. It is commonly used in diet drinks, some brands of chewable vitamin supplements, many sugar-free chewing gums and many other commonly available processed foods including yoghurts.

spartame is also one of the sugar substitutes used by people with diabetes and those trying to lose weight.

Also avoid saccharine. Remember that refined or artificial sugars are found in almost all processed foods.

- The following sweeteners are the best to use:
  - barley malt – good for weight loss, and for people who have diabetes or hypoglycaemia
  - raw unrefined cane or beet sugar
  - raw honey
  - blackstrap molasses, which is rich in essential nutrients including iron and other minerals
  - brown-rice sugar, another good sweetener for people with diabetes
  - stevia and other herbal sweeteners.

FOOD FACTOR 9 – SUPPLEMENTS

If you follow our diet, you should receive all the vitamins you require and you should not need any synthetic supplements. The only supplements that we recommend are natural substances that are likely to contain nutrients in a form more accessible to your body (bio-available).

There is concern that food produced by conventional farming will be lacking in minerals. Nevertheless we recommend against man-made supplements. Instead, we recommend consuming as much organically produced food as possible, with some seafood to provide the minerals needed for good health. Some minerals, when consumed as inorganic man-made supplements, can cause damage: for example copper and iron tablets can block the absorption of other trace elements and cause a cascade of free radicals that can damage DNA, fat and protein and have other unpleasant side effects. Anyone who has ever taken iron tablets will know that they cause constipation. Calcium and magnesium tablets tend to release their alkaline metals too soon and neutralise stomach acid so that the digestive enzyme pepsin cannot begin to break down protein. This can cause problems ranging from acid reflux to poor digestion of proteins. Moreover, if the stomach is too alkaline, bacteria such as *Helicobacter pylori* and *Clostridium difficile* can survive, instead of being killed off in the stomach's natural acid bath. When calcium and magnesium are taken in natural foods, however, they are carried through to the intestine where they are released in appropriately alkaline conditions and taken into the bloodstream.

Guidelines

- Follow the Japanese rule of eating at least thirty different ingredients a day.
- Try to ensure that you consume adequate quantities of the key nutrients in a bio-available form, so that a significant proportion can be absorbed by the body without causing damage. This is especially true of nutrients such as calcium, magnesium, potassium, iron, boron, cobalt, copper, iodine, manganese, selenium and zinc, all of which have important roles in maintaining health.
- Buy organically produced food, from soils rich in organic matter and hence richer in nutrients.
- Eat lots of fresh or lightly cooked vegetables, fruit (including berries), nuts, seeds and seaweed, as well as fish and shellfish.
- Have some brewer's yeast and good-quality kelp every day (follow the instructions on the packet or bottle and ensure you take the correct dose). Brewer's yeast is a good source of B-complex vitamins and minerals such as chromium and zinc, while kelp is a good source of iodine. Both are widely available in health food shops.
- Eat spices, because many have useful levels of trace minerals.
- Have some balanced 3, 6, 9 vegetable omega oils.
- Cod-liver oil is a good source of omega-3 fatty acids, but ensure it is an ultra-pure form such as that manufactured by Seven Seas. Do not have too much, because high levels of the fat-soluble vitamins can accumulate in the body and cause health problems.
- Strict vegans may need to take a good-quality selenium supplement, but be careful not to take too much. They may also need to take vitamin B12, vitamin D, too, if their skin is not exposed to adequate amounts of ultraviolet sunlight.

FOOD FACTOR 10 – HEALTHY DRINKS

Sources of water are problematical, especially in cities. In the past, most people would have drunk fresh water from wells, springs or rivers. Unfortunately, the only way of providing people in large urban centres with adequate water now is to recycle it by treating or reprocessing sewage. During treatment, water is filtered through progressively finer material to remove particles, microbes and chemicals, and it is often mixed with other water to dilute harmful chemicals, so that their concentration falls below legal limits. Reprocessed drinking water can contain concentrations of harmful chemicals including phthalates from soft plastics, breakdown products from detergents and plastics, and pharmaceutical residues including those from the female contraceptive and hormone-replacement pill, all of which are endocrine-disruptors. In some places in the UK, 100 per cent of male fish downstream of sewage discharge are feminised. Reprocessed drinking water can contain many other harmful chemicals, including cancer-causing organic chemicals such as benzene, pesticides and disinfection by-products. Moreover, the presence of pharmaceuticals that can have biological effects at very low concentrations is being reported from water-supply sources in Europe and the USA. Nevertheless, we do not recommend mineral water, especially from plastic bottles, which can release chemicals such as phthalates. Some contain such high levels of radioactivity, nitrates and/or other pollutants that they would be illegal if they came out of a tap. We filter our water through charcoal in a jug, which removes most of the harmful organic substances, and then boil it before drinking.

Guidelines

- Filter tap water through charcoal, then boil it and store it in glass bottles.
- Try to drink liquids stored in glass with cork or aluminium seals, but not in plastic bottles.
- Substitute herbal teas such as camomile, fennel, peppermint, clover and green tea for black tea and coffee (which are high in caffeine). A study of women aged 36 to 45 found that those who drank two cups of coffee a day suffered a net calcium loss

of 22mg per day. Reducing this to one cup daily reduced the loss to just 6mg daily.

- Drink lots of freshly made vegetable and fruit juices from organic produce.
- Do not drink too much alcohol, though the occasional organic cider, real ale or quality (preferably organic, vegan) wine is fine.

A FINAL COMMENT

All this might sound a bit daunting, but when you have adjusted, and are preparing and eating the great meals described here, we believe you will be a convert for life – especially when your health and appearance begin to improve. Anyway, we have done all the hard work of selection for you. All you need to do is make the delicious meals described here to help prevent or treat the condition you are concerned about.

Some people may be able to make all the changes in their diet immediately; others may wish to do this in a series of steps. Priorities may depend on their illness. For example, in the case of high blood pressure, quickly reducing the levels of salt and other sources of sodium and saturated fat may be the highest priority, whereas to prevent or overcome breast cancer or prostate cancer the most important first step in introducing the Plant Programme is to eliminate all dairy produce.

Before looking at particular illnesses, we shall look at the health-giving properties of some foods traditionally used for healing.

Food as Medicine

Over the past half-century or so, we have largely neglected the use of foods and herbs as medicine in favour of pharmaceuticals. There is now renewed interest in the well-documented, nontoxic and inexpensive properties of food in the prevention and treatment of a range of chronic diseases. In the following list we describe the reputed health benefits of some of the whole foods that we use liberally in our recipes.

Alfalfa. Alfalfa (lucerne) is a legume which is a rich source of vitamins and other nutrients, including vitamin A, vitamin B1, vitamin B6, vitamin C, vitamin E, vitamin K, folic acid, calcium, potassium, phosphorus, magnesium and zinc. It helps to lower cholesterol and prevent blood clotting and anaemia. It is used to prevent and treat insulin-dependent type-1 diabetes in South Africa. It is useful in stimulating the growth of connective tissue, in arthritis, for example. A natural laxative, it is thought to be protective against breast cancer because it is rich in phyto-oestrogens. It is also used to treat digestive problems, weight loss, ulcers, kidney and bladder problems, prostate conditions, asthma and hay fever. Traditional Chinese medicine uses alfalfa root to reduce fever, improve urine flow, and treat jaundice, kidney stones and night blindness.

Aloe vera. Aloe vera gel has been used for centuries as a sunscreen by desert Arabs, and it helps to alleviate burns resulting from radiotherapy (but use the gel straight from the plant, rather than man-made creams, which may contain preservatives). It can also be consumed to treat indigestion and stomach ulcers.

Aniseed. Aniseed is anti-parasitic. It contains phyto-oestrogens and therefore helps against breast cancer. It is a medicinal plant recommended for curing nervous asthenia, migraines, vertigoes, rheumatism, cough, bronchial asthma, gastric pains and slow digestion.

Apple. According to the latest research, the old saying, 'An apple a day keeps the doctor away', is fact, not just folklore. Apples contain both insoluble and soluble fibre, which improves bowel movement and reduces the risk of colorectal cancer and diverticulitis. One medium (140g/5oz) unpeeled apple provides more than 10 per cent of recommended daily fibre intake, lowering cholesterol levels and so reducing the risk of hardening of the arteries, heart attack and stroke.

Flavonoids, the pigments that help to give apples their colour, have been shown to help reduce the risk of heart disease. Apple skin and onions are the two major food sources of a potent flavonoid called quercitin. Quercitin is a powerful antioxidant, especially in combination with vitamin C (also found in apples), helping to boost the body's immune system as well as neutralising free radicals (which can damage DNA). Apple fructose, a simple sugar, is broken down slowly, especially with the high fibre in apples, thus helping to keep blood-sugar levels stable. Apples work in a dose-dependent manner: the more you eat, the more protection you get from cancer, heart disease, asthma and type-2 diabetes. Eating apples has also been found to help weight loss. Apples are mildly antibacterial, antiviral and anti-inflammatory. *Caution:* the juice can cause diarrhoea in children.

Apricot. Apricots are a rich source of betacarotene, lycopene, vitamin C and fibre, as well as containing useful amounts of tryptophan – the precursor of mood-boosting serotonin. Both betacarotene and lycopene help fight heart disease and protect against several types of cancer. The vitamin A in apricots – a powerful antioxidant – helps to prevent free-radical damage to the lenses of the eyes, which can lead to cataracts or damage the blood supply to the eyes causing macular degeneration. Apricots are a good source of fibre, helping to prevent constipation and digestive problems such as diverticulosis. For the greatest health benefits, eat fully ripened fruit.

Artichoke (Jerusalem). Since ancient times, the Jerusalem artichoke has been used for liver, bladder and gall-bladder conditions, and for cleaning the blood. The artichoke is high in fibre, potassium, calcium, iron, phosphorus and other important trace minerals. It helps lower blood cholesterol, supports the treatment of hepatitis, arteriosclerosis and gout, and improves gall secretions. It can lower blood sugar moderately and improve the appetite and digestion. It is considered to be a good replacement for potato in diabetic diets. It is diuretic and may help migraine.

Asparagus. Asparagus has been used from ancient times as a medicine, mainly owing to its diuretic properties. It was cultivated by the ancient Egyptians, Greeks and Romans. It is a good source of fibre, B vitamins, folic acid, vitamin C, calcium, iron, magnesium, phosphorus, potassium, zinc, manganese and selenium, and of glutathione, which lowers cancer risk. It is still used to treat urinary-tract infections, as well as kidney and bladder stones and ankle swelling related to heart problems. It is used against parasites in Chinese medicine. Ingestion of asparagus can aggravate gout, however, because it contains high levels of purines.

Avocado. Avocados have the highest protein content of any fruit, and also provide good fats, especially monounsaturated oleic acid (like that in olive oil), which helps to reduce levels of bad LDL cholesterol. They also contain carbohydrate, betacarotene, vitamin E, glutathione and fibre. They help to protect against heart disease, stroke and cancers. The pulp in avocado has antibacterial (against gram-positive bacteria, especially *Staphylococcus aureus*) and antifungal properties. Dieters tend to shun avocados because they are highly calorific (300 calories per fruit), but their high content of nutrients and high protein content mean they are good as part of a weight-loss diet and as baby food.

Banana (and plantain). Bananas contain three natural sugars – sucrose, fructose and glucose – so eating one is a good way of getting a rapid energy boost safely, which makes them popular with athletes. They are also a good source of fibre, protein, potassium, phosphorus, iron, magnesium and vitamins A and B6. They are high in B vitamins, which help to calm the nervous system, and they also contain tryptophan, which the body converts into serotonin, helping you to relax, while lifting your mood and warding off depression. The vitamin B6 in bananas regulates blood glucose levels, which can affect your mood, especially before periods, and can help avoid morning sickness. As excellent brain foods, bananas have been shown to help children through examinations. They can also help when we are stressed, because at such times our metabolic rate rises, reducing our potassium levels.

The potassium in bananas helps to normalise the heartbeat and increases the supply of oxygen to the brain (used in American astronauts' diet to prevent rapid heartbeat). The high potassium and low sodium content makes them good for lowering blood pressure and reducing the risk of stroke. They also stimulate the production of haemoglobin in the blood, helping to treat anaemia. Part of a traditional Jamaican treatment for stomach ulcers, bananas have a natural antacid effect and reduce irritation by coating the lining of the stomach: it is better to eat a banana than pop antacid pills for most cases of heartburn. They are also antibiotics and good laxatives.

The inside of a banana skin rubbed on the skin reduces the swelling and irritation caused by mosquito bites, and it is claimed that the same treatment can remove warts.

Barley. Barley is a traditional heart medicine in the Middle East. It is high in antioxidants, fibre, calcium, potassium, iron and magnesium. It is also high in an enzyme that slows ageing. It is used to treat a range of illnesses including high cholesterol, heart disease, cancer, diabetes and hypertension. Barley water is still used to treat urinary-tract problems, as well as soothing and calming bowel problems.

Beans (legumes, including navy, black, kidney, pinto and soya beans, and lentils). Beans are very high in fibre. They are a powerful treatment for lowering cholesterol. They are an excellent food for diabetics because they help to regulate blood-sugar levels. Populations living on a diet high in beans tend to have lower rates of cancer. Young broad beans contain natural L-dopa, which is converted in the brain to the neurotransmitter dopamine, of value to patients with Parkinson's disease. *Caution:* beans can cause flatulence.

Beets. Beets are good sources of complex carbohydrates, fibre, B vitamins, folic acid, vitamin C, calcium, iron, magnesium, phosphorus, potassium, selenium, zinc and silicic acids. They are a rich source of the element boron, which plays an important role in the production of human sex hormones and may give rise to the reputation of beet as an aphrodisiac. Betaine is important for cardiovascular health and acts with folic acid and vitamins B6 and B2 to reduce levels of homocysteine, which can cause heart disease, stroke and peripheral vascular disease. Beetroot may also help protect against liver disease, caused by alcohol abuse, protein deficiency or diabetes. It also helps individuals with abnormally low levels of stomach acid, which can cause digestive problems. Beetroot juice has been shown to lower blood pressure and thus help prevent cardiovascular problems. Dietary nitrate in beetroot is thought to be a source of nitric oxide, which is used to send signals to the muscles. Beets are among the best foods for relieving constipation and for preventing and treating obesity. Betanins are used as red food colorants, to improve the colour of, for example, tomato paste, sauces, desserts, jams and jellies, ice cream, sweets and breakfast cereals.

Blackberry. The blackberry has been used as medicine since ancient times. The ancient Greeks, for example, used it for gout and the Native Americans for stomach problems. Blackberries (followed by strawberries) have some of the highest levels of phyto-oestrogens, which are thought to protect against breast cancer. They have a high tannin content, which helps to alleviate minor bleeding, diarrhoea, intestinal inflammation and haemorrhoids. They are also used for sore throats, mouth irritations and ulcers. They are among the top ten foods for antioxidants, such as anthocyanin pigments (responsible for their purplish-black colour) and lycopene, as well as vitamins C and E, and ellagic acid; all of these are thought to protect against cancer and other chronic diseases. Blackberries are a natural source of salicylate, the pain killer also found in aspirin. They are a good source of soluble fibre, such as pectin. It is also claimed that they strengthen blood vessels, protect eyesight and reduce the risk of heart disease and age-related disorders.

Blackcurrant. The blackcurrant has an extremely high vitamin C content, good levels of calcium, magnesium, potassium, phosphorus, iron and vitamin B5, and a broad range of other essential nutrients. Other phytochemicals inhibit inflammation linked to heart disease, cancer, microbial infections or neurological disorders such as Alzheimer's disease. Blackcurrant-seed oil is also rich in gamma-linolenic acid (GLA), an essential fatty acid. Blackcurrants are used to treat rheumatic conditions and gout, and as a nerve tonic.

Blueberry. Blueberries are very high in antioxidants and are a good source of vitamins C and E, manganese and fibre, yet very low in calories. They are high in natural aspirin. They help to neutralise damage by free radicals to the collagen matrix of cells and tissues, which can lead to cataracts, glaucoma, varicose veins, haemorrhoids, peptic ulcers, heart disease and cancer. They have been shown to be particularly protective against oxidative stress affecting the eye and brain, and are therefore considered helpful against macular degeneration and Alzheimer's disease. They are antiviral and antibiotic. They block bacteria attaching to the lining of the urinary tract, where they cause infection. They also help curb diarrhoea.

Broccoli. Broccoli is antiviral. Like other cruciferous vegetables, it contains antioxidants, including quercetin, glutathione, betacarotene, indoles, vitamin C and sulphoraphane, which help treat cancer, including that of the lung, colon and breast. It speeds up removal of oestrogen from the body and is therefore particularly helpful in suppressing breast cancer. It is rich in cholesterol-reducing fibre and helps to protect against ulcers. It is an excellent source of chromium, which helps regulate insulin and blood sugar. *Caution:* cooking can destroy some of the antioxidants and it is best eaten raw or lightly cooked, except for those with hypothyroidism.

Brussels sprouts. The Brussels sprout is a cruciferous vegetable with similar anti-cancer and oestrogenic activity to broccoli and cabbage. It is rich in antioxidants and indoles.

Cabbage (including bok choy). Cabbage is rich in vitamins A, B, C and E, and contains high levels of iron and sulphur. It is claimed that the leaves, after pounding, can relieve joint pain and breast pain associated with breast feeding. It is also a member of the cruciferous vegetable family. It is antibacterial and antiviral. Used in ancient Rome as a cancer cure. It contains many anti-cancer and antioxidant compounds. It speeds up oestrogen metabolism, and is thought to help block breast cancer and suppress growth of polyps, which can develop into colon cancer. It helps protect and treat stomach cancer and ulcers. Raw cabbage, including in coleslaw, is better for health except for those with hypothyroidism. *Caution:* cabbage can cause flatulence. Some of its important components are destroyed by cooking.

Carrot. Carrots are an excellent source of vitamins A, B, C and K, and of folate, potassium, manganese, molybdenum, phosphorus, magnesium and soluble fibre (which helps to lower cholesterol levels and prevent constipation). They are an excellent source of antioxidant compounds, and the richest vegetable source of the pro-vitamin A carotenes (vitamin A is essential for vision, including night vision – providing some factual basis for the Second World War legend that eating carrots helps you to see in the dark). Carrots' antioxidant compounds help to protect against cardiovascular disease and cancer, including lung cancer in smokers. The betacarotene in carrot protects arteries and helps to prevent strokes and alleviate angina. They protect against macular degeneration and the development of senile cataracts, the leading causes of blindness in the elderly. Cooking makes it easier for the body to absorb betacarotene from carrots.

Cauliflower. Cauliflower is a member of the cruciferous vegetable family. It contains many of the same anti-cancer and hormone-regulating substances as broccoli and cabbage. It is best eaten raw or lightly cooked, but not by those affected by hypothyroidism.

Celery. Celery is a rich source of vitamin K and has useful amounts of folate and vitamins A, B and C, as well as potassium, molybdenum, manganese, calcium, magnesium, tryptophan, phosphorus, iron and fibre. It is low in calories. It is useful for giving a salty flavour to soups and stews to avoid adding salt. Celery contains several other active compounds that promote health, including phthalides, which may help to lower cholesterol levels, and coumarins, which may be useful in cancer prevention. Celery's potential for reducing high blood pressure has long been recognised by Chinese medicine practitioners, and Western scientists have recently attributed this to the phthalides it contains, which can help relax the muscles around arteries as well as reducing stress hormones, which cause blood vessels to constrict. The potassium, calcium and magnesium it contains have also been associated with reduced blood pressure. It also helps lower cholesterol by increasing bile secretion.

Celery has a long and prestigious history of use as a medicine. It is rich in potassium and sodium, the minerals most important for regulating fluid balance by stimulating production of urine. The ancient Greeks used wild celery seeds as a diuretic. Compounds in celery called acetylenics have been shown to stop the growth of tumour cells. *Caution:* eating celery before or after vigorous exercise can induce mild to serious allergic reactions in some people.

Chilli pepper. Chilli pepper is antibacterial and antioxidant. It is especially good for the respiratory tract as it acts as a decongestant, helping to prevent bronchitis and emphysema. It also helps to prevent stomach ulcers. Paprika made from hot chilli peppers is high in natural aspirin and is useful in treating headaches and joint pain. Chilli pepper speeds up the metabolism, helping to treat obesity. It also helps to dissolve blood clots. Most of chilli pepper's activity is attributed to capsaicin, the substance that makes it taste hot. This substance also makes prostate-cancer cells commit suicide; tests showed that capsaicin triggered 80 per cent of the cells to start the process leading to cell death. The same research showed that tumours treated with capsaicin were smaller. *Caution:* there is some evidence that a high consumption of chilli peppers is associated with stomach cancer.

Cinnamon. Cinnamon is an ancient spice, used for thousands of years. It is a good source of manganese, fibre, iron and calcium. Studies have shown that just half a teaspoon of cinnamon per day can lower LDL cholesterol, and it also has an anti-clotting effect on the blood so it helps protect against heart attacks and strokes. Take cinnamon on your porridge every day, and you may be able to avoid having to take statin pills. Several studies suggest that cinnamon helps to regulate blood sugar, so it is helpful for people with type-2 diabetes. It has also been shown to reduce the proliferation of leukaemia and lymphoma cancer cells. Half a teaspoon of cinnamon powder combined with a tablespoon of honey every morning before breakfast has been shown to relieve arthritis. In some studies, cinnamon has been shown to stop medication-resistant yeast infections. When added to food, it inhibits bacterial growth and food spoilage, including *E. coli* bacteria in unpasteurised juices, making it a natural food preservative. One study found that smelling cinnamon boosts cognitive function and memory.

Clove. Cloves came originally from the Maluku Islands (formerly known as the Moluccas, or the Spice Islands), part of Indonesia. Remains of cloves have been found in a ceramic vessel in Syria dating from 1721BC, and later they were highly prized by the Romans. Cloves contain useful amounts of calcium, iron, magnesium, phosphorus, potassium, zinc, copper, manganese and selenium, as well as vitamins A, C and B and folate. Their main active ingredient, eugenol, is an anti-inflammatory and helps to treat rheumatic disease. They are used in Ayurvedic medicine (they are called *lavang* in India), in Chinese medicine and in Western herbalism and dentistry, where the essential oil is used as a painkiller for dental emergencies. Cloves are used to increase hydrochloric acid in the stomach and to improve peristalsis, and are also said to be a natural de-worming agent. In Chinese medicine, cloves (known as *ding xiang*) are used to treat hiccups and fortify the kidney. They are also used in formulas for impotence and to clear some types of vaginal discharge, for morning sickness, together with ginseng and patchouli, and for vomiting and diarrhoea due to spleen and stomach coldness. Clove oil is used to treat various skin disorders such as acne. It is used to treat severe burns and skin irritations, and to reduce the skin sensitivity. In the West, cloves and clove oil are used for dental pain, and to a lesser extent to reduce fever, as a mosquito repellent and to prevent premature ejaculation. Clove may reduce blood-sugar levels. *Caution:* large amounts of cloves should be avoided in pregnancy, and they should be avoided by people with gastric ulcers, colitis or irritable bowel syndrome. In overdoses, cloves can cause changes in liver function. Excessive use of the oil can cause kidney damage. If in doubt, consult a medical herbalist.

Coriander. Coriander is both a herb and a spice, since both its leaves and its seeds are used. Fresh coriander leaves are also known as cilantro. The Persians cultivated it over three thousand years ago. It is rich in vitamin C, betacarotene, calcium and phosphorus. Research suggests that it may be beneficial for lowering blood cholesterol and for lowering blood-sugar levels, so it is of value in treating hypoglycaemia and diabetes. It also contains an antibiotic substance, dodecenal, which can prevent *Salmonella* food poisoning and gastroenteritis. In addition to dodecenal, eight other antibiotic compounds have been isolated from fresh coriander.

Cranberry. Cranberries are a good source of vitamins C and K, and of potassium. They are antiviral. Native people have used cranberry to treat urinary-tract infections and other illness for centuries. Modern research has shown that the berries contain proanthocyanidins, which inhibit adhesion of bacteria, including antibiotic-resistant strains of *E. coli*, to the urinary tract epithelium, and hence they can be used to prevent and fight such infections. Another substance in cranberries has been shown to reverse and inhibit the action of the oral bacteria responsible for dental plaque and periodontal disease and to help prevent and treat stomach ulcers by inhibiting the adhesion of the *H. pylori* bacterium to human gastric mucus and epithelium. In addition to ulcers, *H. pylori* infection has been linked to stomach cancer, acid reflux disease and gastritis. Cranberries are very high in antioxidants, and research suggests that they protect against atherosclerosis (the accumulation of LDL (bad) cholesterol, in arteries, restricting blood flow and increasing blood pressure and predisposing people to heart disease and stroke). They are also high in salvestrols, which help to prevent and treat cancer.

Cucumber. Cucumber was used in the ancient civilisations of Egypt, Greece and Rome, not only as a food but also for its beneficial skin-healing properties. It is still used topically for various types of skin problems, including swelling under the eyes, sunburn and dermatitis. The flesh of cucumbers is composed mainly of water and is particularly low in calories, but it also contains ascorbic acid (vitamin C) and caffeic acid, which help to soothe skin irritations and reduce swelling. The outer dark green skin is rich in fibre, silica, potassium and magnesium, and contains some tryptophan. Cucumber juice is often recommended as a source of silica to improve the skin. Traditionally cucumber has been used to treat fevers, constipation, skin eruptions, high blood pressure, rheumatism, obesity and acidosis. It is a mild diuretic and helps treat irritation of the urinary tract.

Cumin. Cumin is a traditional Indian remedy for indigestion, which is, perhaps, why it is included in many curry powders. It is an excellent source of iron, which is a key component of haemoglobin, several important enzyme systems involved in energy production and metabolism, and the immune system. Iron is also a co-factor in the synthesis of serotonin from tryptophan. Cumin is also a good source of manganese. According to some Indian traditions, it is not taken during pregnancy.

Date. Dates are an important part of the Muslim tradition and are traditionally eaten to break the fast after Ramadan. In the Qur'an it says that when the mother of Jesus was giving birth to him and was experiencing pain, she was told, 'Shake the trunk of the palm towards you and fresh, ripe dates will drop down onto you.' Scientific studies confirm that eating dates is beneficial for pregnant women because they contain substances that strengthen the muscles of the womb. They have a high content of healthy sugars, protein, fibre, vitamins A and B and folate, as well as some vitamin C, E and K. They are an excellent source of calcium, iron, magnesium, phosphorus and potassium. They are also a good source of the trace elements zinc, copper, manganese and selenium. Dates have been important in sustaining desert people for centuries. They are reported to be useful in the treatment of respiratory disorders, heart conditions, cancer, anaemia, allergies and constipation. Bedouin Arabs, who eat dates regularly, have low incidence rates of cancer and heart disease. High in natural aspirin. It is a good natural laxative. Dried fruits, including dates, are linked to lower rates of certain cancers, especially pancreatic cancer. *Caution:* dates contain compounds that may cause headaches in some people.

Eggplant or aubergine. Aubergine contains substances called glycoalkaloids, which have been used topically to treat some types of skin cancers. Eating eggplant may lower blood cholesterol and counteract other detrimental effects of fatty food. Eggplant also has antibacterial and diuretic properties.

Fennel. Fennel has been grown around the Mediterranean Sea and the Near East since ancient times. It is still an important part of the healthy Mediterranean diet, especially that of Italy. The bulb is an excellent source of vitamin C, dietary fibre, potassium, manganese, folate and molybdenum. Fennel is also a good source of niacin, phosphorus, calcium, magnesium, iron and copper. It contains a combination of beneficial phytonutrients, which are powerful antioxidants. One of these, anethole, has been shown to reduce inflammation and help prevent cancer by shutting down signalling mediated by the tumour necrosis factor. Fennel oil has been shown to protect the liver from toxic chemicals in animal experiments. The high fibre content of the fennel bulb helps reduce cholesterol levels and protect against colon cancer, and the high levels of folate help to protect against dangerous homocysteine, which can directly damage blood vessels and is a significant risk factor for heart attacks and stroke. Its high levels of potassium also help to lower high blood pressure. Fennel contains phyto-oestrogens, which are protective against breast cancer. It aids digestion and is a soothing diuretic. It also helps to prevent blood clotting.

Fenugreek seed. Fenugreek is a spice common in the Middle East. Has anti-diabetic properties, helping to control surges of blood sugar and insulin. It is also anti-diarrhoeal, anti-ulcer and anti-cancer. It helps to lower blood pressure and prevent intestinal flatulence.

Flaxseed and flaxseed oil. Flaxseed and the oil derived from it are used mainly to treat constipation and inflammation of the digestive tract, including gastritis and colitis. They lower levels of blood fat and bad LDL cholesterol, both of which are associated with heart attacks and strokes. Flaxseed reduces harmful blood cholesterol levels because of its soluble fibre. It helps to prevent colon and breast cancer. It improves mood, diminishes allergies and promotes healthier skin.

Fig. Fig is a laxative, with anti-ulcer, antibacterial and anti-parasitic properties. It helps to prevent cancer. *Caution:* figs cause headaches in some people.

Fish (oily) and fish-liver oil. These are high in omega-3 oils, which protect against heart attacks and strokes. They can relieve the symptoms of rheumatoid arthritis, osteoarthritis, asthma, psoriasis, high blood pressure, Raynaud's disease, migraine headaches, ulcerative colitis and, possibly, multiple sclerosis. The oil is an anti-inflammatory agent and anticoagulant. It raises levels of good HDL cholesterol and lowers triglycerides in the blood. It helps to protect against glucose intolerance and hence type-2 diabetes. Some fish are high in antioxidants, such as selenium and coenzyme Q-10. The oil has anti-cancer properties, especially against colon cancer and breast cancer. Fish high in omega-3 fatty acids include sardines, mackerel, herring, salmon and fresh tuna. Unfortunately, many dangerous man-made chemicals are fat-soluble and bio-accumulate in fatty fish, so limit your consumption. Some of the benefits of fatty fish are obtained by eating marine plankton and algae, which is where the fish obtain their omega-3 fatty acids.

Garlic. Garlic has long been used to treat many types of illness. It is a broad-spectrum antibiotic, antiviral and anti-intestinal-parasitic, which boosts the immune system generally. It lowers blood pressure and blood cholesterol and helps to prevent blood clotting and heart attacks. It contains many antioxidants and is number one on the US National Cancer Institute's list of cancer-preventive foods. A good treatment for colds, it acts as a decongestant, expectorant, anti-spasmodic anti-inflammatory agent. It helps to relieve flatulence and diarrhoea. It is oestrogenic and a diuretic. It is considered to lift mood, with a mild calming effect. Eat garlic both raw and cooked. *Caution:* more than three cloves a day of raw garlic can cause flatulence, diarrhoea and fever in some people.

Ginger. Ginger is an antibiotic and antioxidant, and may help to treat cancer. Ginger is a traditional ingredient of herbal medicine, as an aid to the absorption of other ingredients. It is used to treat nausea, vomiting (including that caused by morning sickness, travel sickness and sickness associated with chemotherapy), headaches, chest congestion, cholera, colds, diarrhoea, stomach ache, heart disease, rheumatism, cold hands and feet, hiccups and nervous diseases. It helps prevent migraine headaches and treat osteoarthritis and the symptoms of rheumatoid arthritis. It acts as an anti-thrombotic and anti-inflammatory agent and may protect against ulcers.

Grape. Grapes are rich in antioxidants. Grapes and grape-seed oil help prevent blood clotting and maintain good HDL cholesterol levels in blood. Red grapes (but not white or green grapes) are high in the antioxidant quercetin. Red grapes may be antibacterial and antiviral. Grape-seed oil is high in polyunsaturated fat and raises good HDL cholesterol, so it is good for patients with coronary heart disease. There is some evidence that grapes may contain anti-ageing chemicals.

Grapefruit. Grapefruit pulp (but not the juice) contains a substance that lowers blood cholesterol and helps to clear clogged arteries. It contains anti-cancer substances that are particularly protective against stomach and pancreatic cancer. The juice is antiviral and high in various antioxidants, especially vitamin C.

Honey. Honey is antibiotic, with sleep-inducing, sedative and tranquillising properties. *Caution:* it is high in sugar, so it should be used sparingly. Use only raw, not processed honey. There is evidence that locally produced honey, which contains traces of pollen from nearby vegetation, can reduce hay fever because taken orally it reduces the sensitivity of the eyes and nose.

Kale. Kale is another member of the cruciferous vegetable family. It contains anti-cancer chemicals, including betacarotene, lutein and indoles. It helps to regulate the body's oestrogen.

Kiwi fruit. Kiwi fruit is used in Chinese traditional medicine to treat stomach and breast cancer. It is high in vitamin C.

Lemon. Lemon has traditionally had many therapeutic uses. Lemon juice is a natural antiseptic, which can be applied safely directly to cuts, bruises and skin infections. Lemon juice is good for asthma, headaches, pneumonia and arthritis. Lemon helps to treat coughs, colds, influenza and the onset of fevers generally. It is a mild diuretic. The juice also helps the removal of some drug residues from the body. *Caution:* do not use where there are inflammatory conditions of the digestive tract.

Liquorice. Liquorice is antibacterial. It is considered to have anti-cancer properties, and helps to prevent and treat ulcers and diarrhoea. It may act as a diuretic. Only real liquorice has these properties, not confectionary flavoured with anise. *Caution:* too much liquorice can raise blood pressure. Also, it should not be taken by pregnant women.

Maize. Maize has antiviral and anti-cancer properties. It contains phyto-oestrogens. *Caution:* it is a common cause of food intolerance linked to symptoms of rheumatoid arthritis, irritable bowel syndrome, headaches and migraine-related epilepsy in children.

Melon (pink, green and yellow, such as cantaloupe and honeydew). Melon helps to prevent blood clotting. It contains the antioxidant betacarotene, folic acid and other vitamins.

Mushroom (Asian, including shiitake). Mushroom is used to treat heart disease and cancer in Asia. Mushrooms such as maitake and shiitake help prevent and/or treat cancer, viral diseases, such as influenza and polio, high blood cholesterol, blood clotting and high blood pressure. A compound in shiitake mushrooms is a broad-spectrum antiviral agent that aids immune function. No therapeutic effects are known for the commonly available button mushroom. Indeed, it has been claimed that this type of mushroom has the potential to initiate cancer unless cooked.

Mustard (including horseradish). Mustard contains up to 30 per cent protein. Leaf mustard contains calcium, phosphorus, magnesium and vitamin B, and mustard seeds are a very good source of selenium and omega-3 fatty acids. They are also a good source of phosphorus, magnesium, manganese, dietary fibre, iron, calcium, protein, niacin and zinc. Mustard has been used medicinally since ancient times, and mustard seed is mentioned in the New Testament. It stimulates appetite and digestion, increasing saliva. It is a powerful expectorant and decongestant, helping to break up mucus; it can clear the sinuses as effectively as many commercial products. It is claimed that it increases metabolism, burning off extra calories and thus helping to treat obesity. Mustard increases blood circulation, hence its use as mustard plaster to increase blood flow and promote healing following sprains and similar injuries. The sulphur in mustard is helpful as a paste in treating skin problems. Mustard helps to lower blood pressure. It is also antibacterial, antifungal and antiseptic, and has anti-inflammatory properties so it can help ease the symptoms of rheumatic diseases. Isothiocyanates in mustard have been shown to inhibit the growth of cancer cells in the digestive tract in animals. *Caution:* like all other cruciferous plants, mustard contains goitrogens – naturally-occurring substances that can interfere with the functioning of the thyroid gland – so mustard is best avoided by those with an underactive thyroid.

Nuts. Nuts have anti-cancer and heart-protective properties. Nuts generally are high in antioxidant vitamin E, which is protective against chest pain and artery damage. Nuts, including peanuts, are also good regulators of insulin and blood sugar, preventing steep rises, making them good foods for those with glucose intolerance and diabetes. Peanuts are oestrogenic. Walnuts and almonds help reduce cholesterol and contain high concentrations of oleic acid, a monounsaturated fat, similar to that in olive oil, which is known to protect arteries from damage. Walnuts contain ellagic acid, an antioxidant and anti-cancer substance, and are also high in omega-3 type oil. Brazil nuts are extremely rich in selenium, an antioxidant linked to lower rates of heart disease and cancer, but they can be naturally radioactive. *Caution:* nuts are a major cause of acute allergic reactions in susceptible individuals.

Oats. Oats contain protein. They are an excellent source of manganese and a very good source of selenium. In addition, they are a good source of vitamin B1, vitamin E, magnesium, phosphorus, zinc, copper, iron and manganese. They are also a good source of soluble and insoluble fibre. Insoluble fibre speeds the passage of stools through the gut, relieving constipation. Soluble fibre breaks down as it passes through the digestive tract, forming a gel that reduces the absorption of cholesterol into the bloodstream. The soluble fibre in oats can reduce bad LDL cholesterol without lowering good HDL cholesterol, and protects against heart disease generally. According to the American Cancer Society, the cancer-fighting properties of insoluble fibre are also due to its ability to destroy toxic bile acids and to its content of anti-cancer phytochemicals. Oats also slow down the digestion of starch, making it beneficial to diabetics, and help to stabilise blood sugar. They help fight anxiety and insomnia, and were the treatment for hyperactivity in children before the advent of drug treatments. *Caution:* oats contain purines, which can lead to excess accumulation of uric acid and thus aggravate gout and the formation of kidney stones in certain individuals. Large quantities can cause flatulence.

Olive oil. Olive oil lowers bad LDL cholesterol without lowering good HDL cholesterol, helping to protect arteries from plaque. It reduces blood pressure and helps to regulate blood sugar. It has powerful antioxidant properties and is the best, most stable oil for cooking.

Onion (including chives, shallots, spring onions and leeks). Onion is anti-inflammatory, antibiotic, antiviral. It is reputed in some ancient civilisations to cure a wide range of diseases. It contains exceptionally strong antioxidants and other anti-cancer agents. Shallots and yellow and red, but not white, onions, are the richest dietary source of the powerful antioxidant quercetin, which is also a sedative. Onion thins the blood, lowers cholesterol, raises good HDL cholesterol and reduces blood clotting. It also helps to treat asthma, chronic bronchitis, hay fever, diabetes, atherosclerosis and many types of infection. There is evidence that onions and leeks contain substances that support good gut bacteria. It has been suggested that damage to gut bacteria by the use of antibiotics or pollutants can cause ill health. *Caution:* onions can aggravate heartburn and may promote flatulence.

Orange. Orange is a natural cancer-inhibitor. It contains carotenoids, including betacarotene, terpenes and flavonoids. Its high content of vitamin C may help prevent asthma attacks, bronchitis, breast cancer, stomach cancer, atherosclerosis and gum disease. *Caution:* it may aggravate heartburn.

Papaya. Papaya contains papain, which assists in the digestion of protein. It helps digest gluten. It is widely used as a contraceptive in India and Sri Lanka, because it interferes with the activity of progesterone, the hormone essential in maintaining pregnancy. *Caution:* for this reason it should not be eaten by pregnant women.

Parsley. Parsley is an excellent source of vitamins A, C and K, and a good source of iron and folate. It is rich in volatile oil components such as myristicin, limonene, eugenol and alpha-thujene, and in antioxidant flavonoids, which help mop up free radicals (which are linked to cancer, heart disease and ageing). Its volatile oil components have been shown to inhibit tumour formation in animal models, particularly in the lungs. They also help to neutralise carcinogens like benzopyrenes in cigarette and charcoal-grill smoke. Parsley is a good source of folic acid, which helps to convert dangerous homocysteine (which, at high levels, can directly damage blood vessels) into benign substances, reducing the risk of heart attack and stroke. Folic acid is critical for proper cell division. It is particularly important for cancer prevention in the colon and the cervix, because they have rapidly dividing cells. *Caution:* it contains oxalates, which may cause problems in some people.

Peppers. Peppers belong to the colourful *Capsicum* genus, which includes sweet peppers (known as capsicums, bell peppers or green/red peppers, depending on where you live) and the spicy chillies, which contain capsaicin (see under **Chilli pepper**, above). Besides lots of vitamin C, sweet peppers also provide vitamin B6, phytochemicals such as lycopene and betacarotene (the precursor of vitamin A), folate, potassium and lots of fibre. Peppers help to fight off colds, asthma, bronchitis, respiratory infections, cataracts, macular degeneration, angina, atherosclerosis and cancer.

Pineapple. Pineapple is antibacterial and antiviral. It contains an antibacterial enzyme called bromelain, which is anti-inflammatory. Pineapple aids digestion, is used in treating rheumatoid arthritis, helps dissolve blood clots, and is good for preventing osteoporosis and bone fractures because of its high manganese concentration and alkali-generating properties. It is also mildly oestrogenic. It promotes digestion of proteins. *Caution:* ensure you always clean your teeth well after eating pineapple because it can affect their roots.

Plum. Fresh plums contain lots of vitamin C, and both fresh plums and their dried form (prunes) are good sources of fibre and potassium. They also contain powerful antioxidants, which help to protect fats in the body, including those in cell membranes. They are antibacterial and antiviral. Prunes are a partiularly good natural laxative; they are high in fibre, sorbitol and natural aspirin.

Potato. Potatoes originated in the Andes, where they are thought to have been cultivated for between 4,000 and 7,000 years, providing a staple food crop for people living at these high altitudes. They are a very good source of vitamin C (they were used on Spanish ships to prevent scurvy), and are also a good source of vitamin B6, copper, potassium, manganese and fibre. Their content of phenolic antioxidants is similar to that of broccoli, spinach and Brussels sprouts. They contain substances known to protect against cardiovascular disease, respiratory problems and certain cancers, as well as quercetin and kukoamines (also found in goji berries), which help to lower blood pressure. They contain phyto-oestrogens.

Pumpkin. Pumpkins and their seeds were a celebrated food of Native Americans, who valued them both as food and for their medicinal properties. Pumpkins are rich in iron, zinc and fibre, and the flesh is very high in carotenoids (including betacarotene), which neutralise free radicals that can attack cell membranes and are linked to ageing, cancer and heart disease. They are also high in the antioxidants lutein and zeaxanthin, which scavenge free radicals in the eye, helping to prevent cataracts and macular degeneration.

Pumpkin seeds are a very good source of phosphorus, magnesium and manganese and a good source of zinc, iron, copper and vitamin K. They also contain protein. They help to fight prostate and bladder problems and help with muscular-skeletal problems because they contain anti-inflammatory substances, without the side effects of anti-inflammatory drugs. They are used in many cultures to treat tapeworms and other parasites. They are high in phytosterols, which have been shown to reduce levels of LDL cholesterol and protect against many cancers. They also contain L-tryptophan and other useful compounds that can help against depression.

Raspberry. Raspberries are an excellent source of fibre, manganese and vitamin C, and also a good source of vitamin B2, folate, niacin, magnesium, potassium and copper. In addition, they contain significant amounts of the antioxidant anti-cancer phytochemical ellagic acid. They are antiviral and high in natural aspirin. Raspberries are also a rich source of flavonoids, such as quercetin, which give the fruit their red colour and their powerful antioxidant and antimicrobial properties, including the ability to prevent overgrowth of certain bacteria and fungi, including the yeast *Candida albicans*. Eating a diet which includes lots of antioxidant fruits such as raspberries can help protect against eye problems, such as cataracts and macular degeneration. *Caution:* raspberries contain oxalates, so people with kidney or gallbladder problems may want to avoid eating them.

Rice. Rice has anti-diarrhoea and anti-cancer properties. Like other seeds, it contains anti-cancer protease inhibitors. Of all the grains and cereals, it is the least likely to provoke flatulence or intolerances that can aggravate bowel problems. Rice bran is an excellent treatment for constipation. It also lowers cholesterol and helps to prevent kidney stones developing.

Seaweed, including kelp (brown or laminaria-type seaweed). Kelp and other seaweeds are rich sources of soluble fibre (which helps protect against heart disease and stroke), calcium, sodium, magnesium, potassium, iodine, iron, zinc and trace elements such as lithium (which can be deficient in typical Western diets), as well as vitamin A (as betacarotene), the B vitamins, folic acid and trace amounts of vitamin B12 (which rarely occurs in land vegetables). Seaweed also contains vitamin C. Chinese sailors, since before the time of Admiral Zheng He (1421) always ate sea vegetables, as well as growing their own vegetables on ship, and hence never suffered from scurvy. The sea vegetables such as arame, hijiki, kombu and wakame, which are high in alginic acid, bind with any heavy metals in the intestines and carry them out of the body as faeces. Seaweed is antibacterial and antiviral. It kills the herpes virus, for example. One of the best foods for treating hypothyroidism. Kelp may also lower blood pressure and cholesterol. Wakame boosts immune functioning. Nori kills bacteria and seems to help to heal ulcers. A chemical from wakame seaweed helps to prevent blood clots. Most types of seaweed have anti-cancer activity.

Soya. Soya is rich in phyto-oestrogens, which help menopausal problems. It has anti-cancer properties and is thought to be particularly helpful in preventing and treating breast cancer, possibly one reason why rates of breast and prostate cancers are low among the Chinese and Japanese, who traditionally consume soya as part of the diet. Soya beans are the richest source of potent protease inhibitors, which have anti-cancer and antiviral properties. Soya beans lower blood cholesterol substantially and may help to prevent kidney stones. Lecithin, an antioxidant, is high in soya beans. It is good for the nervous system and helps to improve memory. It emulsifies fat in the blood and protects cells against oxidative damage. It also helps to maintain a healthy liver and heart.

Spinach. Spinach is an excellent source of antioxidants and anti-cancer substances, including betacarotene and lutein. It is rich in fibre, which helps to lower blood cholesterol. *Caution:* some of its antioxidants are destroyed by cooking, so eat it raw or lightly cooked.

Strawberry. Strawberries have antiviral and anti-cancer properties. *Caution:* strawberries can contain very high amounts of pesticide contaminants, so eat only organically grown fruits.

Sweet potato (also known as yam in the USA). Sweet potatoes are a good source of dietary fibre, betacarotene, vitamin C, vitamin B6, iron and calcium. They help protect the cardiovascular system, because vitamin B6 helps to destroy homocysteine, which can directly damage blood vessel walls.

Tea (including green, oolong and black tea; not herbal teas). Tea has diverse pharmacological activity, mainly due to catechins. It is antibiotic and antiviral. Tea acts as an anticoagulant, protects arteries, helps to prevent and treat ulcers and protects against tooth cavities. It has anti-diarrhoeal and diuretic properties. Green tea has well-documented anti-cancer properties. Tea drinkers appear to have fewer damaged, clogged arteries and fewer strokes. Green tea, popular in Asian countries, is highest in catechins, followed by oolong and black tea. *Caution:* excessive tea drinking can aggravate anxiety, insomnia and symptoms of PMS because of its caffeine content and it can also promote the development of kidney stones because of its high oxalate content.

Tomato. Ignore all the nonsense from wacky practitioners suggesting that tomatoes are bad for health. If any practitioner or book says this – find another one! In fact, tomatoes are an excellent source of vitamins C, A and K. They are also high in boron, copper, molybdenum, iron, potassium, magnesium, manganese, phosphorus, dietary fibre, protein, chromium, folate and vitamins B1, B2, B3, B5, B6 and E. A carotenoid called lycopene found in tomatoes is a powerful antioxidant and helps to prevent DNA damage associated with ageing, cancer and heart disease. Studies in humans have shown lycopene to be protective against many cancers, including colorectal, prostate, breast, endometrial, lung and pancreatic cancers, especially when eaten with fat-rich foods such as avocado, olive oil or nuts because carotenoids are fat-soluble and are absorbed with fats.

The latest research suggests that it is not just lycopene but also the combination of nutrients in tomatoes that make them so good for health. The fibre and potassium in tomatoes also help to reduce bad LDL cholesterol levels and blood pressure, and there is new evidence that lycopene helps prevent blood clotting in diabetics and others.

Oxidative stress associated with free radicals and increased levels of inflammatory compounds such as TNF-alpha have been linked to many chronic degenerative diseases, including atherosclerosis, cardiovascular disease, cancer, osteoporosis and Alzheimer's disease. Consumption of tomato juice or gazpacho soup has been shown to decrease the levels of these inflammatory compounds by about a third.

Forget all the nonsense about purple tomatoes to persuade us to eat genetically modified (GM) foods. It is the deepest-red organic tomatoes and products such as organic ketchup that contain the most lycopene – more than non-organic produce. Always choose the deepest-red organic tomatoes, ketchup, tomato sauce, juice and other tomato products, and buy products that use whole, not peeled, tomatoes.

Turmeric. Turmeric is one of the most important medicinal spices. Its main active ingredient, curcumin, which gives turmeric its intense cadmium-yellow colour, is an anti-inflammatory agent as powerful as cortisone and helps to relieve the symptoms of rheumatoid arthritis. It lowers cholesterol, helps to prevent blood clotting, protects the liver, protects the stomach against acid, lowers blood sugar in diabetics, and has powerful anti-cancer properties.

Watermelon. Watermelon contains lycopene and glutathione, which have antioxidant and anti-cancer properties. It is also mildly antibacterial, and helps to prevent blood clotting.

Wheat. Wheat is anti-parasitic. Whole wheat, particularly wheat bran, is high in fibre and is one of the best natural laxatives. The bran has strong anti-cancer properties, including against colon cancer. *Caution:* it is a common cause of food intolerances and allergies, giving rise to symptoms of rheumatoid arthritis, irritable bowel syndrome and neurological illnesses in some individuals.

Yam. Yams are a good source of dietary fibre, potassium, vitamin C, manganese and vitamin B6. They do not contain oxalates, purines or goitrogens, so are safe for most people. They help protect the cardiovascular system, because vitamin B6 helps to destroy homocysteine, which can directly damage blood vessel walls, while their high levels of potassium help to control blood pressure. Dioscorin, a storage protein contained in yams, may also help reduce hypertension. Yams also contain diosgenin, which is chemically similar to progesterone and has been shown experimentally to affect hormonal patterns in animals.

Chinese herbal medicine has traditionally used wild yam to support the female endocrine system – during lactation, for example. There is no firm research evidence to support the claim that yam helps to ease menopausal symptoms, but there is much anecdotal evidence that wild yam cream used topically is helpful.

Illnesses: Prevention and Treatment with Food

This section of the book suggests some ways in which you can modify your diet to prevent, treat and overcome some common diseases. Since food and the way it is digested are fundamental to understanding how diet can help to prevent and treat disease, you may wish to turn first to pages 100–103, where the digestive system is explained.

ALLERGIES AND INTOLERANCES TO FOOD

What is the disease?

An allergy is an inappropriate response by the body's immune system to a substance not normally harmful. The immune system is a highly complex defence mechanism that helps fight infections, but in some people it wrongly identifies a nontoxic substance as a problem and overreacts so that the allergic response becomes the disease itself. Substances that cause allergic reactions are called allergens. Here we are dealing specifically with food allergies, but other common allergens include pollen, dust, mites and moulds, cosmetics and cleaning agents, some metals, animal hair, insect bites and some antibiotics.

A food allergy or hypersensitivity is an abnormal response to a food triggered by the immune system. In true food allergies, two parts of the immune response are involved; one is an antibody that circulates in the blood, the other is a type of cell called a mast cell. These cells occur in all body tissues, but especially the nose, throat, lungs, skin and gastrointestinal tract – the typical sites of allergic reaction. The food protein fragments responsible for an allergic reaction are not broken down by cooking or by digestion; hence in some people they can cross the gut wall into the blood, causing allergic reactions, which in some cases can be serious. In the most extreme cases such reactions can cause serious (anaphylactic) shock that can lead to death.

In the case of food intolerances, many people have flatulence or other unpleasant reactions to something they eat. This can be due to a lack of the enzyme needed to digest the food and is not a true allergic response, which is why it is called 'food intolerance'. Lactose (milk sugar) intolerance is very common, especially among non-Caucasians. This is a particular concern since lactose is used as a filler or base for many prescription and herbal tablets. Gluten intolerance is also common (see details under **Coeliac disease**, page 105).

It is worth remembering that many foods contain preservatives, emulsifiers, colorants and other additives (for example, benzoic acid (E120) and sulphur dioxide), which may be the source of the allergy rather than the food itself. Sulphites are commonly used to preserve food and prevent discoloration, and may be used in wines, salad bars and frozen foods. They often cause allergic reactions. Check ingredients carefully for any ingredients ending in sulphite, and, if purchasing salad from a salad bar, ask whether any sulphites have been used to preserve the appearance of the food.

What causes it and who does it affect?

In the case of true food allergies, the problems arise when a particular food is digested for the first time and tiny protein fragments stimulate the body to produce the antibody against the food, which then attaches to the surface of mast cells. The next time that food is eaten, the antibody on the mast cell triggers the release of chemicals such as histamine that produce the allergic reaction.

Serious allergies, including food allergies and allergic drug reactions, now affect as many as one in ten people in Western countries. No one knows why some people develop allergies to certain substances. Although people in their late teens and early twenties are most likely to suffer allergies, they can develop at any age.

Some allergies are thought to have a genetic component. People most likely to develop food allergies will probably have a family history of hay fever, asthma or eczema. Allergic symptoms in children can include runny noses, wheezing, coughing, ear infections, rashes and stomach upsets. Hippocrates (the father of Western medicine) and Dr Spock (the influential twentieth-century paediatrician) swore by milk-exclusion diets for children. In a recent study a significant proportion of a group of infants diagnosed with cow's milk allergy were still highly allergic at the age of ten.

Food intolerances other than lactose and gluten intolerance are less well understood or documented, though there is anecdotal evidence that the number of people affected has increased.

Some intolerances are more prevalent in particular ethnic groups, lactose intolerance among non-Caucasians being one example.

What are the main symptoms?

The timing and location of the allergic reaction depend on factors such as individual digestion. If the chemicals are released in the nose and throat, the allergy will be reflected by an itching tongue or mouth and in serious cases people may have difficulty breathing (including developing asthma) or swallowing. If the cells are in the gastrointestinal tracts the symptoms will include vomiting and diarrhoea or abdominal pain. In severe cases such allergies can cause such a severe drop in blood pressure that it causes death. On the other hand, if the chemicals reach the skin, the allergy will produce hives or intense itching. The onset of any of these symptoms can vary from a few minutes to an hour or two.

Recently, we helped a young man with serious hives who, after waiting for six months, had been seen by a National Health Service consultant who prescribed antidepressants – which made the problem worse! Guess what? We tracked down his problem to preservatives in white bread, and the antidepressants he had been prescribed contained the same preservative. Since we identified the source of his problem he has been free of his skin condition.

Other symptoms of allergies and intolerances can be less clearly identified with food, and include problems with mood changes (including depression), watery itchy eyes and blurred vision, and swelling of parts of the body.

How is it diagnosed?

A good doctor will use very pure substances to carry out skin tests to diagnose allergies, either on the forearm or the back. In the case of food allergies and intolerance, however, this method may not work. Some intolerances and allergies, like gluten intolerance, can be picked up by a blood test, but others require an exclusion diet and/or a full and accurate food diary to identify the food that is causing problems. The best method of diagnosis is to work with your doctor by keeping a detailed food diary so that you can examine the types of food consumed and relate the times that a food was consumed to the appearance of symptoms. If you suspect a food, for example wheat, you should take some pure wheat grain rather than bread (which can contain other substances) to check if this is the source of the problem. However, many food intolerances may be difficult to find this way. Elimination diets are often needed, beginning with foods unlikely to cause problems – classic examples being pears and lamb. Suspect foods are then introduced into the diet one by one until the problem is identified; the foods that are most likely to cause problems, such as wheat and dairy, are introduced last.

What is the conventional medical treatment?

Conventional medical practitioners may prescribe steroids and/or antihistamine medications, but these merely mask the symptoms and they can have serious side effects, especially if used over the long term. We recommend identification and exclusion of the allergen or the food that is causing the intolerance.

What are the foods involved?

Over 170 foods have been documented as causing allergic reactions. Most sufferers are affected by the so-called 'big eight': dairy products, eggs, soya, wheat, peanuts, shellfish, fruit and tree nuts. Other common sources include bananas, beef products, chocolate, citrus fruit, oats, salmon, strawberries, tomatoes and white rice. Processed and refined foods can cause allergies and intolerances, and many people are allergic to food colouring. Many people on the Plant Programme diet have reported to us that their symptoms have disappeared after following our diet, although people affected by soya allergies should use rice, oat or pea milk to replace dairy. Those with intolerances to wheat and gluten-based cereals will find lists of suitable and unsuitable foods on pages 108–109.

ANXIETY AND DEPRESSION

We find it helpful to distinguish anxiety, which involves hyperactivity, worrying and repetitive thinking – a condition which we nickname 'the Lady Macbeth syndrome' – from depression, which is associated with lethargy, loss of interest and general feelings of worthlessness. In some cases people may have elements of both: indeed, Jane has suffered from them both. These conditions have been suggested to indicate problems with the brain's neurotransmitters (chemical messengers that carry messages across nerve synapses). Anxiety can be caused by problems with the GABA neurotransmitter (and often accompanies benzodiazepine withdrawal), while depression is often caused by deficiency in the serotonin neurotransmitter. Since the prime mode of action of many insecticides is to block neurotransmitters, and several are specifically targeted at blocking GABA, it is important to have as much organically produced food as possible. See also Jane's book co-authored with Janet Stephenson, *Beating Stress, Anxiety and Depression*.

ANXIETY

What is the disease?

Anxiety can be either acute or chronic. Acute anxiety normally involves panic attacks, when the body's natural 'fight or flight' reaction occurs inappropriately, and results from the body producing too many stress hormones, especially adrenaline and cortisol. This, in turn, causes the body to increase its metabolic rate to produce large quantities of energy. Muscles tense and heartbeat and breathing rates increase, while the composition of the blood changes, making it more likely to clot. This type of reaction has survival value in dangerous situations, but at other times the symptoms associated with the adrenaline surge can be distressing and frightening. Hyperactivity in children may be a form of this condition.

Chronic anxiety is a milder form, with most sufferers feeling a low-level sense of anxiety most of the time. The commonest symptoms are headache and chronic fatigue, and some people may suffer occasional panic attacks.

What causes it and who does it affect?

The most likely food factors are considered to be pesticide residues in food, the use of food additives such as tartrazine, a lack of essential nutrients such as omega-3 fatty acids in the diet and in some cases alkalosis caused by an unbalanced diet.

Anxiety is a far more common problem than was once thought and can affect people from their teenage years into old age. It appears to affect twice as many women as men, but this may reflect the fact that men are less likely to acknowledge or report that they have such problems. Panic attacks are thought to be caused when the brain sends and receives false emergency signals.

In some cases anxiety seems to run in families and may be linked to a relatively harmless abnormality of heart function.

What are the main symptoms?

Symptoms of acute anxiety in panic attacks include shortness of breath, feelings of claustrophobia and lack of air, heart palpitations, chest pain, dizziness and feeling very hot or very cold, sweating and nausea. Such panic attacks can occur at any time and last for between a few seconds and thirty minutes, though it may seem much longer to the sufferer. They can occur in response to foods contaminated with pesticides, and to certain foodstuffs themselves, drugs, illness and/or stress. Food allergies and hyperglycaemia (low blood sugar) are common in those affected.

Symptoms of chronic anxiety include generalised pain and aching, muscular twitching and stiffness, insomnia, nightmares and early waking, decreased libido and inability to relax.

How is it diagnosed?

It is usually diagnosed after physical causes of symptoms have been eliminated and on the basis of a careful case history. Blood levels of stress hormones such as adrenaline and cortisol may be measured and the adrenal glands may be scanned, because they can be enlarged in those subject to chronic stress. It has been suggested that an increased level of stress hormones, as a result of their overproduction by the body, underlies such conditions as 'shell shock'.

What is the conventional medical treatment?

In the past, conventional medicine tended to use benzodiazepines such as Valium and Librium to treat the condition or, where there was a component of depression, tricyclic antidepressants. Various psychological treatments may be used, including counselling to try to release pent-up emotions and psychotherapy to try to analyse underlying causes. Cognitive behavioural therapy (CBT) is now frequently the preferred treatment. These methods are expensive, and waiting lists on the NHS tend to be long. Frequently people are required to pay for private treatment.

In acute attacks, patients are asked to breathe into paper bags so that the carbon dioxide they breathe out is reabsorbed, helping to acidify their blood. This provides an important clue to one factor in anxiety.

Children may be prescribed drugs such as Ritalin.

What are the foods involved?

We emphasise that it is important to have organically produced food, not only fruit and vegetables but also meat and fish to avoid insecticide and worming residues, which target the GABA neurotransmitter in the brain. Another factor in anxiety can be an excess of alkali-producing foods in the diet. Our treatment is based on helping people to adjust their diet to reduce alkalosis, which is known to cause anxiety symptoms. (See chart on pages 28–29, showing acid- and alkali-producing foods; ensure that you are not eating too many foods from the top left of the diagram without balancing them with adequate amounts of acid-forming foods.) Porridge is the old treatment for hyperactivity in children. It contains beneficial neuroactive chemicals and it helps to acidify the blood quickly. It is still used by herbalists to overcome anxiety symptoms induced by benzodiazepine withdrawal symptoms. It is also helpful in dealing with insomnia, so have your porridge at night before retiring to bed. We have given this tip to people with insomnia, including people affected by 'restless leg syndrome', and they have all reported significant alleviation of their symptoms without any of the adverse side affects associated with taking sleeping pills.

High-protein foods promote the production of dopamine and norepinephrine (often known as noradrenaline in the UK) which, in turn, promote alertness and make us think and act more quickly; these may be unhelpful in anxiety states.

The brain is largely composed of fat, and one of the problems with the modern Western diet is thought to be imbalance of omega-3 and omega-6 fatty acids. Food supplements that are helpful in restoring the balance of fatty acids that our brains need include ultra-pure cod-liver oil (make sure you buy only the ultra-pure varieties as the others can contain cancer-causing chemicals) and virgin cold-pressed organic balanced omega 3, 6 and 9, vegetable oils, which include flax, hemp, sesame and pumpkin, evening primrose and rice-bran oils (follow the instructions for dosage on the packet).

In summary, follow the basic Plant Programme, maintaining a 60 per cent alkali-forming to 40 per cent acid-forming foods ratio, and also do the following:

- Eat foods high in Taurine, the precursor of GABA, including meat and fish (dairy and eggs are poor sources of Taurine; there is none in plant foods).
- Make sure that you have enough magnesium in your diet. Spinach, beans, seeds and nuts are good sources.
- Take brewer's yeast tablets; these contain B vitamins, which help to reduce anxiety and calm the nerves.
- Take kelp tablets; these contain iodine, calcium and magnesium, which help brain function and relieve anxiety and nervousness.
- Start the day with some ultra-pure cod-liver oil.
- At lunchtime have some balanced omega 3, 6, 9 vegetable oils.
- Before going to bed, have some organic porridge oats with a little raw brown sugar and soya milk.

Other tips

- Try to avoid taking benzodiazepine as sleeping tablets or tranquillisers, since these work by causing the brain to overproduce GABA, so that a vicious circle can be set up. If you are already dependent on this drug, try to reduce your dosage in a series of steps.
- Yoga and/or pilates can be extremely helpful, by regularising breathing and hence blood chemistry.
- Never use insecticides. Many of them are fat-soluble, and if they come into contact with the skin they can travel, via nerves, to the central nervous system and affect neurotransmitters.
- Meditation may be helpful.

DEPRESSION

What is the disease?

Globally, more working days are lost through depression than any other illness, and it is one of the most serious health threats worldwide.

The two main types of depression are unipolar and bipolar. Patients affected by bipolar disease alternate between depression and mania so the disease is frequently called manic depression. Here, we are concerned mainly with unipolar types of depression. This is characterised by episodes that frequently recur several times during a person's life. The commonest type is chronic low-level depression which is not completely disabling but does prevent people from functioning normally and interferes with social interaction.

What causes it and who does it affect?

Depression is one of the commonest medical problems in most developed countries. In Britain, one in ten people are depressed, and they may have anxiety as well. In the USA, people born after the Second World War are twice as likely to develop the illness, and the age of onset is falling. An article in the *New Scientist* pointed out that it was far more common in affluent countries, and this was attributed to the composition of fat in the diet: people in developing countries consume a much higher proportion of omega-3 fatty acids. Other factors may be the much lower use of pesticides and other man-made chemicals in these countries.

Neurotransmitters are extremely important in mood and behaviour. Low levels of serotonin, for example, can lead to depression, anxiety and sleep disorders.

Depression can affect people of all ages, from the young to the elderly, and is reported to be twice as common in women as in men. It affects the nervous system, especially moods, thoughts and behaviour, and can affect the whole body, including causing a loss of appetite and inducing sleeplessness. The causes of depression are not fully understood but factors are thought to include stress (such as a traumatic life event), chemical toxins or imbalances in the brain, thyroid disorders, poor diet, lack of exercise, or serious illnesses such as glandular fever. It is commonly caused by food allergies and intolerances, especially coeliac disease, low blood sugar or diseases of the digestive tract, all of which prevent absorption of key nutrients. Hypothyroidism is another possible cause of depression. It seems likely that there is some genetic link to depression, too: up to 50 per cent of people suffering from recurrent depression will have had one or more parents affected by the condition.

A poor diet, especially one with lots of junk foods and fizzy drinks, which contain many chemical additives, is a common cause of depression or can make symptoms worse because it affects the levels of neurotransmitters, which are closely linked to mood. One of these, serotonin, is thought to play a key role in mood, sleep and appetite, with low levels leading to depression and sleeping disorders.

What are the main symptoms?

Symptoms can last for weeks, months or years, and include a loss of interest in anything and an inability to experience pleasure. Other symptoms include chronic fatigue, sleep disturbances including excessive sleeping, changes in appetite and digestive disorders, headaches, backache, and feelings of worthlessness and inadequacy. In extreme cases, people may consider suicide. People with depression frequently withdraw from any contact with friends and family, and focus only on their own troubles. They show symptoms that can range from appearing angry and irritable to sad and despairing or they may show little or no emotion. They may also be lethargic and despondent.

How is it diagnosed?

Usually by taking a detailed case history. New techniques of brain scanning, which can identify problems in brain chemistry, are being introduced. Biochemical tests on blood or urine samples can also be carried out.

What is the conventional medical treatment?

Normally a patient is given drug treatment, depending on the type of depression and the views of the physician. Some people may be treated with talking therapies such as counselling, psychotherapy or cognitive therapy (see further under **Anxiety**). In extreme cases they may be treated with electroconvulsive therapy (ECT).

What are the foods involved?

Too much acid-generating food that causes acidosis is a key factor in depression. We have helped two people to improve their mood by persuading them not to live only on cheese sandwiches made with refined white bread. Eating complex carbohydrates helps to increase serotonin production and thereby helps depression.

As well as keeping closely to the Plant Programme and eating plenty of raw or lightly cooked fruit and vegetables, soya products, whole grains, seeds, nuts, millet and legumes, you should follow these guidelines:

- Eat foods high in tryptophan, the precursor of serotonin, including meat (especially turkey), soya protein (such as tofu), barley, sweet potatoes, mangoes, legumes, papaya and nuts (especially cashew nuts and peanuts).
- Avoid diet drinks and products containing artificial sweeteners such as aspartame, which have been suggested to block the formation of serotonin.
- Avoid foods high in saturated fats such as chips and hamburgers that can cause poor circulation, including to the brain.

- Eat unrefined complex carbohydrates, which increase serotonin production in the brain, which in turn improves mood. Before eating more wheat, though, make sure you do not have coeliac disease, since this can make matters worse.
- Avoid refined sugars; use only the sweeteners recommended in Food Factor 8, page 42.
- Avoid or limit alcohol and caffeine intake.
- Avoid processed foods and soft drinks, which can contain a wide range of additives, many of them linked to behavioural problems and some them described as neurotoxins.
- Investigate the possibility that food allergies are contributing to your state of mind by keeping a food diary and trying an elimination diet (see further under **Allergies and intolerances to food,** page 72).
- Take brewer's yeast to ensure adequate levels of vitamin B and essential trace elements such as chromium.
- Take kelp tablets, which contain iodine, calcium and magnesium, which help brain function and relieve anxiety and nervousness.
- Take cod liver oil for omega-3 fatty acids, but make sure it is the ultra-pure variety.
- Take balanced omega 3, 6, 9 oils, but ensure you buy them in a glass bottle and that they are organically produced.
- Have porridge at night to help with sleeplessness.
- Some people find St John's wort can ease depression and improve mood, but it takes up to four weeks to begin to have an effect and you should discuss its use with your doctor, especially if you are on prescription medication.
- Ginkgo biloba has been found to be helpful.

Other tips

- Exercise, especially outdoor exercise, is particularly helpful, so a good long walk or a cycle ride in the sunshine may help.
- Keep a food diary to detect any correlation between your mood and the foods you eat.
- Consider joining a support group.
- Meditation may be helpful.

AUTOIMMUNE DISEASES

Many diseases, including type-1 diabetes and multiple sclerosis (MS), have been suggested to be autoimmune diseases, whereby the body's immune system, which is meant to protect it against pathogens and other assaults, systematically attacks the body's own tissues, leading to a progressive loss of physical and/or mental function. Rheumatic fever is well known to be an autoimmune disease, whereby the body produces antibodies to destroy streptococcus bacteria but these antibodies also attack heart muscle because its protein is so similar to that of the bacteria. Some doctors suggest that diseases such as MS and rheumatoid arthritis may be the result of a similar process in relation to organisms in the facial sinuses and gut, but there is little scientific evidence to support these theories.

Any theory on the cause of such conditions must explain why many show similar clinical characteristics, and why they are often found together in the same populations. It must also explain why they are more common at high latitudes. The incidence of MS in Scandinavia, for example, is more than 100 times that near the equator. Migration studies show a pattern for these conditions whereby, depending on the age at which people move to a new country, the incidence of the disease changes to that of the local host community within one or two generations.

According to Professor T. Colin Campbell the term 'autoimmune diseases' includes rheumatoid arthritis, pernicious anaemia, MS, type-1 diabetes and lupus erhythematosus. Other authors include many other conditions in the autoimmune group, including schizophrenia. Campbell suggests that, like cancer, they are in fact all one disease, with different symptoms depending on which part of the body is affected. Campbell points out that one of the foods that supplies foreign proteins that mimic human proteins is dairy milk. The casein in milk is an extremely large, complex molecule that is difficult for humans to break down, especially if their digestion is impaired, for example if they do not have enough stomach acid or their stomach pH is too high as a result of taking antacids or calcium pills.

According to Campbell, 'the breadth and depth of evidence implicating cow's milk as a cause of type-1 diabetes is overwhelming.' Moreover, studies in twenty-four countries show a relationship between consumption of cow's milk and the incidence of MS that is virtually identical to that between cow's milk consumption and type-1 diabetes. Studies of autoimmune diseases in relation to nutrition show an increased risk with the consumption of animal-based foods – especially cow's milk – though factors such as viruses, lack of sunlight, consumption of saturated fats and low intakes of omega-3 fatty acids are also factors.

About 3 per cent of people in the US (about one in thirty people) suffer from an autoimmune condition. Approximately two and half times as many men as women are affected.

The treatment of autoimmune diseases is typically with immunosuppressant drugs, medication to reduce the immune response. Early results suggest that stem-cell therapy may arrest, or in some cases reverse, damage caused by autoimmune response – in multiple sclerosis, for example. We shall consider some of the treatments further in the sections that follow.

CANCER

This disease can affect almost any part of the body, most commonly the epithelial cells which line organs and the body cavity.

What is the disease?

Cancer is a general term for more than a hundred diseases characterised by the unusual and uncontrolled division of abnormal cells in a part of the body. Solid tumours in the breast or colon, for example, can invade and destroy surrounding normal tissue. Cancer cells can also spread via the lymph system and bloodstream to form secondary cancers in other parts of the body by a process known as metastasis.

What causes it and who does it affect?

The body is constantly making new cells to replace old worn-out ones by a process called mitosis, which is designed to make an exact copy of the cell being replaced. If a fault is introduced in the genes controlling mitosis, cancer can result.

The three main sets of genes involved in mitosis, and hence in the development of cancer, are the ones instructing the cell to grow and divide and begin mitosis (proto-oncogenes), those that tell it to stop doing so (tumour suppressor genes), and those that, if there is a mistake, tell the cell to fix it up or commit suicide (apoptotic genes). The fact that just a tiny subset of genes, out of the more than 25,000 genes in the human genome, are damaged in cancer cells explains why it is so difficult to treat and cure the disease.

Cancer is now considered to involve three stages: initiation, promotion and proliferation (see Figure 2). Initiation is thought to give rise to a cell that is the ancestral cell to the cancer. This can be inherited in the case of rare cancers, such as a type of childhood cancer of the eye called retinoblastoma, but more commonly initiation reflects damage caused by environmental factors. Damage to DNA leading to an initiated cancer cell can be caused by viruses, bacteria, fungi, ionising radiation or carcinogenic chemicals. Normally, except in the case of inherited cancer, the body repairs such a cell or tells it to commit suicide. Promotion, however, appears to favour initiated cells with their damaged genes that control cell growth and division relative to normal cells. Substances called growth factors are increasingly implicated in this stage of the development of cancer and in the proliferation of the disease through the body.

It is thought, if current trends continue, that by 2020 cancer will affect one in three people at some time in their life, although rates differ greatly for different types of cancer and in different parts of the world. The rates of reproductive cancers such as breast cancer and prostate cancer have risen markedly in the West. Breast cancer is now the most frequently diagnosed cancer in women in the USA, with 213,000 new cases in 2006. A woman's lifetime risk of developing breast cancer in the USA is now 1 in 8. Prostate cancer shows similar trends and it is set to overtake lung cancer as the number-one cancer affecting men in the next three years – in the USA it already has. The age-standardised incidence of breast cancer in the USA was about 100 cases per 100,000 women, compared with only about 19 in China in the year 2002. The rates for prostate cancer per 100,000 were about 125 compared with about 1.5 respectively in the two countries in the same year.

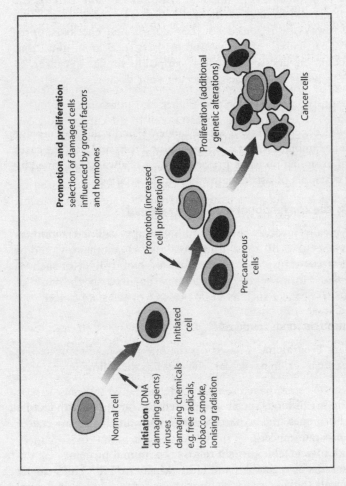

Figure 2 Initiation, promotion and proliferation of cancer cells
Modified from Greenwald, P., Cancer Chemoprevention, *BMJ*, vol. 324, 2002.

What are the main symptoms?

The symptoms vary markedly according to the type of cancer, and can include a lump, bleeding, or symptoms such as a cough in the case of lung cancer. Any unusual symptoms of any part of the body or general feelings of ill health such as sudden weight loss should always be reported to your doctor and checked appropriately, particularly if the symptoms persist. Bear in mind that many common illnesses can cause symptoms similar to cancer, so try not to worry unduly before seeing your doctor.

How is it diagnosed?

Again this depends on the type of cancer. Usually this will involve physical examination, X-rays, scans, blood tests and in some cases internal examination using probes. Cancer is always confirmed by taking a sample of tissue, or biopsy, to be studied.

What is the conventional medical treatment?

This typically involves surgery, radiotherapy and/or chemotherapy in the case of solid tumours, and chemotherapy and/or bone-marrow transplants in the case of blood diseases such as leukaemia. Hormone treatments may be used in the case of reproductive cancer such as breast cancer or prostate cancer.

What are the foods involved?

The Plant Programme is based on the one Jane used to overcome her breast cancer. In particular, the diet has the following features. It:

- eliminates all foods such as dairy, which contain growth factors and hormones (this is particularly significant for breast cancer and prostate cancer);
- is high in vegetable protein relative to animal protein;
- has masses of vegetables and fruit, which are full of anti-cancer chemicals (only one such claim is made for a chemical in animal products – CLA in unhealthy milk fat – and that is a chemical that the cow gets from the plant food that it eats!);
- eliminates refined carbohydrates, which can generate increased levels of growth factors in the body;

- has the right amount of fats – which are all healthy fats;
- recommends fresh organically produced food, which contains live enzymes and other beneficial substances but lower levels of harmful chemicals;
- is high in fibre, to remove toxins from the body;
- is high in essential nutrients.

If you are particularly concerned about cancer, we recommend that you follow the diet suggested here and supplement your repertoire of recipes with the original *Plant Programme* and our book *Understanding, Preventing and Overcoming Osteoporosis.* Choose other ingredients to ring the changes using the section on food as medicine on pages 48–71.

For breast, ovarian or prostate cancer, specifically, see also Jane's books *Your Life in Your Hands: Understanding, Preventing and Overcoming Breast Cancer* and *Prostate Cancer: Understand, Prevent and Overcome.*

CARDIOVASCULAR DISEASE (CVD):
angina, atherosclerosis, heart attacks, heart failure, high blood pressure (hypertension), arrhythmia and strokes

The cardiovascular system comprises the heart, which acts as a strong pump, and a one-way circulatory system that carries blood around the body (see Figure 3). Blood is pumped from the heart through a complex network of arteries, which divide into finer arterials and eventually capillaries. Blood is returned to the heart through capillaries, veinules and veins. Venous blood is generally charged with the waste products of metabolism, including carbon dioxide. Blood is reoxygenated by being circulated through the lungs, to which the pulmonary artery carries oxygen-poor, carbon-dioxide-rich blood. When carbon dioxide has been exchanged for oxygen in the lungs, the pulmonary vein returns the blood to the heart before it is recirculated though the body (see Figure 4).

The heart muscle is crucial to the whole system and, like every other organ in the body, it needs its own blood supply, which is called the coronary circulation. Arteries are thick-walled tubes with a circular covering of elastic fibres containing muscle that

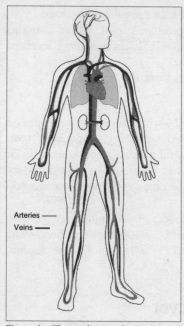

Arteries ———
Veins ——

Figure 3   The cardiovascular system

absorbs the great pressure of a heartbeat and slows the blood down. Veins, unlike arteries, have thin, slack walls because the blood has lost pressure, and the dark, reddish-blue blood of the veins moves sluggishly.

Although the brain is not part of the cardiovascular system, strokes, which affect it as a result of problems with blood supply, are considered in this section.

What is the disease?

CVD includes angina, heart attacks, strokes and other disorders of the heart and blood-vessel system. Despite the introduction of high technology for the diagnosis of heart problems, the first indication of disease may be life-threatening, because disorders are often far advanced before there are any symptoms.

The main process involved in the development of CVD is atherosclerosis or hardening and clogging of the arteries. This commonly affects the coronary arteries, which deliver blood to the heart muscle itself. Clogged arteries are usually associated with plaques of mainly cholesterol but there is now debate over whether the cholesterol is the main problem or whether it is the body's mechanism of putting 'sticking plasters' over blood vessels damaged by another chemical called homocysteine. This can be generated by the metabolism of animal protein such as dairy and red meat if the diet lacks adequate amounts of folic acid. The liver makes cholesterol, which we need for many functions including the production of oestrogen, testosterone, vitamin D and bile, but the amounts consumed by those eating a conventional Western diet mean that levels in the body can be far too high.

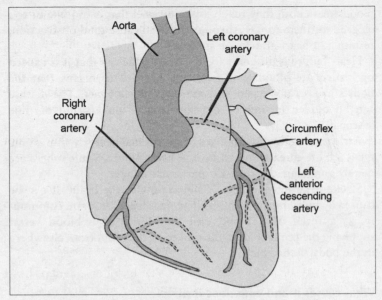

Figure 4 The heart and coronary arteries

Atherosclerosis is the main underlying process involved in the development of **high blood pressure** (hypertension), which is one of the commonest predisposing factors to CVD generally. The condition causes the heart to work harder, wearing down this vital muscle. Untreated high blood pressure may lead to further heart disease and congestive failure, as well as to strokes and kidney failure.

The first symptom of **coronary heart disease** is often **angina**, which causes severe chest pain and occurs when the arteries that supply blood to the heart muscle have become so narrow that there is insufficient oxygen supply. When advanced, coronary artery disease can lead to heart attacks (myocardial infarction, or a 'coronary'). Heart attacks are caused when the coronary arteries become so obstructed that the flow of blood *to* the heart is cut off completely, causing damage to the heart muscle itself. This is most commonly because a blood clot, frequently from elsewhere in the body, causes an obstruction in one or more of the already clogged coronary arteries. Plaques or clots that break off from their blood vessel attachments anywhere in the body move through the bloodstream until they reach a blood vessel that is too fine or too clogged for them to pass through; this can cause total obstruction, resulting in heart attacks or strokes.

Heart failure is different from a heart attack in that it is caused by inadequate blood flow *from* the heart. This means that the body's needs for oxygen and nutrients are not met. The disease can be sudden (acute) or develop over a long period of time (chronic).

Arrhythmias are disturbances of the normal heart rhythm. Some types are life-threatening and cause heart failure, while others are merely annoying and pose no particular danger.

Stroke is an interruption of blood flow to the brain. It can be caused by bleeding in the brain (haemorrhagic) or, more commonly, as a result of a blood clot that forms in a blood vessel supplying the brain or that has moved to the brain from elsewhere in the body (ischaemic).

What causes it and who does it affect?

Until recently, CVD was the number-one killer in the USA, where it is responsible for almost 50 per cent of all deaths. It remains the number-one killer in most other Western countries. At the beginning of the twentieth century, it was not even in the top ten fatal diseases, and in developing countries where people continue to live on simple, low-animal-protein, high-vegetable-protein diets there is still a low incidence of the disease. Many teenagers on Western diets high in burgers, shakes and fries already have fatty streaks in their blood vessel walls and even plaques in their arteries.

Although CVD is traditionally thought of as a disease affecting older men, it is increasing in women, particularly women who have gone through the menopause, and in many Western countries more women die from the disease than from breast cancer and uterine cancer combined. Although common in older people, it is not an inevitable result of ageing. For example, ninety-year-olds in the Hunza society in Kashmir are free of CVD and have normal blood pressure. The role of the Western diet, high in saturated fats, refined carbohydrates and salt, and with nutritional deficiencies, is widely seen to be a major factor in the disease, although stress, obesity, diabetes, smoking, lack of exercise, the use of HRT, and genetic predisposition are also considered important. Kidney disease and disorders of the pituitary, adrenal or thyroid gland can also be an underlying cause of CVD. Heart disease may be caused by certain bacterial or viral infections, or even by some allergies (see page 72).

What are the main symptoms?

High blood pressure may have few symptoms initially, but eventually it causes symptoms such as rapid pulse, shortness of breath, dizziness, headaches and sweating. By the time that symptoms have developed, the condition may be more difficult to treat.

Angina is typically characterised by severe chest pain, usually after physical exertion. The pain goes away or lessens in intensity after resting.

A heart attack typically feels as if someone is applying intense pressure to the chest, causing pain that can extend to the shoulder, arm, neck or jaw, although the amount and type of chest pain vary from one person to another: many people mistake the pain for indigestion. Some sufferers have no symptoms at all.

Symptoms of heart failure include fatigue, ashen skin colour, shortness of breath and accumulation of fluid, especially around the ankles.

The symptoms of strokes are almost always sudden, and include numbness or weakness of the face, arm or leg, usually on one side of the body, confusion or trouble with speaking or understanding speech; difficulty in seeing in one or both eyes; problems with walking; dizziness, loss of balance and/or co-ordination; and severe headaches. Treatment needs to be given quickly: every minute counts.

Small strokes (transient ischaemic attacks) may last for only a few minutes but should never be ignored. They require treatment with drugs or surgery.

How is it diagnosed?

CVD is generally diagnosed by:

• taking blood-pressure measurements and pulse rates;
• examining the heart rhythm using a stethoscope;

- taking blood tests, including measurement of the levels of total blood cholesterol and HDL/LDL cholesterol, triglycerides, homocysteine, sugar and uric acid.

Heart disease is diagnosed by:

- taking an electrocardiogram (ECG), which measures heart rhythm and electrical activity – but this cannot predict problems in advance and shows the problem only after it exists;
- taking chest X-rays, although these have the same problems as ECGs;
- taking an echocardiogram, which uses ultrasound waves to pick up subtler changes in heart muscle and its internal valves;
- angiography, involving injection of a dye to study blood circulation – but this can be risky and expensive.

Strokes are identified by carrying out a Magnetic Resonance Imagery (MRI) brain scan.

Cholesterol and blood-pressure levels

Two important measurements used in assessing cardiovascular health are levels of blood fat (including cholesterol and triglycerides) and blood pressure. The ratio of low-density 'bad' lipoprotein (LDL) to high-density 'good' lipoprotein (HDL) may also be determined. It is possible to buy a machine to measure blood pressure and pulse rate, so you can monitor these indicators yourself.

Table 5 Blood pressure levels

Blood pressure	Good	Normal	Borderline	High
Systolic (when the heart contracts and pumps blood out)	120 or less	121–130	131–140	141 and higher
Diastolic (between beats, when the heart fills with blood again)	80 or less	81–85	86–90	91 and higher

An elevated diastolic pressure is considered more serious than a high systolic pressure.

What are the conventional medical treatments?

Conventional treatment includes specific treatment for underlying causes such as diabetes and may also include anti-hypertensives (ACE) inhibitors, beta-blockers, blood thinners such as aspirin and warfarin, and/or a combination of hydralazine and isosorbide dinitrate, digitalis, nitroglycerin and diuretics depending on the specific CVD condition. Sterols (alcohols derived from plants) are increasingly prescribed for CVD, but they can have side effects. It would seem more sensible simply to eat more fruit and vegetables. Statins are now commonly prescribed. Some of these substances are derived from micro-organisms, while others are their synthetic equivalents. They work by inhibiting an enzyme that is involved in the synthesis of cholesterol.

In some cases surgery may be necessary, including angioplasty, bypass surgery for blocked coronary arteries, valve replacement, pacemaker installation and heart transplantation, depending on the type and seriousness of the CVD.

Doctors always recommend that people with CVD stop smoking and avoid passive smoking. Patients will also be advised to stop taking HRT, avoid excessive alcohol consumption, reduce any stress and obesity, follow an appropriate exercise programme, and to improve their diet, especially to reduce saturated fat and salt intake.

What are the foods involved?

Every major study for many years has shown that CVD is directly related to diets high in saturated fats, including meats (especially red meat), dairy and eggs, whereas a low-saturated-fat diet greatly reduces the risk of these diseases. The heart, in particular, as the most active muscle in the body, requires proper nutrition.

A diet high in animal protein, including dairy and meat, will contain high levels of an amino acid called methionine. If the diet is also too low in food containing folic acid (green leafy vegetables and fruit such as apples and melons), high levels of the cardiovascular-damaging chemical homocysteine can be produced.

Many of the recommendations of the Plant Programme diet will reduce the risk of CVD. These include a:

- low intake of saturated fats and cholesterol;
- low intake of sodium, including salt;
- low intake of processed refined food (including fats and sugars);
- low animal protein relative to vegetable protein;
- low animal protein relative to green leafy vegetables and fruit;
- low intake of refined sugar;
- high proportion of foods with high levels of fibre, including complex carbohydrates (such as whole grains, pulses and seeds), vegetables and fruit;
- high intake of antioxidants to limit damage from free radicals;
- high intake of soya products such as soya milk, tofu and tempeh (instead of dairy) but use only low-salt soya sauce in those of our recipes that include soya sauce.

In addition, other factors of particular relevance to the prevention and treatment of CVD include a diet that is:

- low in hydrogenated fats, contained in many margarines and spreads;
- low in homogenised fat, especially homogenised milk;
- low in pickled or cured foods, especially meats;
- low in chlorinated and/or soft water;
- high in lecithin e.g. avocado, soya;
- high in garlic, onions and cayenne;
- adequate in the levels of oily fish or other good sources of omega-3 fatty acids;
- low in vitamin-K-rich foods such as liver and egg yolks, which can increase blood clotting;
- low in caffeine, which increases heart rate and blood pressure and the risk of heart arrhythmias;
- moderate in alcohol intake.

Choose other fruits, vegetables, herbs and spices that you enjoy and that are protective of the cardiovascular system from the list on pages 48–71.

Other nutrients that are important include minerals, especially selenium, copper, zinc and manganese as well as calcium, magnesium and potassium (but not as pills). Drinking soft water can replace the minerals calcium and magnesium, which are protective against CVD, with sodium, which can increase atherosclerosis and blood pressure. This can be a problem with certain types of water softeners.

DIABETES AND HYPOGLYCAEMIA

What is the disease?

Diabetes is caused by problems with the pancreatic hormone, insulin. This controls the amount of glucose (sugar) in the blood and its absorption into cells, which need it to produce energy. In people with diabetes, glucose accumulates in the bloodstream instead of being taken into and used by the cells. Eventually, high blood-sugar levels can damage blood vessels, leading in turn to eye disease, heart disease, nerve damage to the limbs and other organs, kidney disease, fluid retention, infections (particularly of the mouth, lungs, bladder and genitalia), and skin sores that fail to heal.

There are two main types of diabetes:

- type 1 (insulin-dependent diabetes: diabetes mellitus)
- type 2 (non-insulin-dependent diabetes)

What causes it and who does it affect?

One in twenty of the world's adult population now has some form of diabetes.

Type 1

Five to ten per cent of all diabetics have type 1, which usually starts at an early age. It is considered by many conventional doctors to be an autoimmune disease, whereby the body destroys the insulin-producing cells in the pancreas. This is attributed in some cases to an inappropriate immune response to a viral infection. Although there is probably a genetic predisposition, it has been suggested that the disease is caused by an allergy to bovine protein, fragments of which are incorporated in the insulin-producing cells of the pancreas.

Type 2

Type-2 diabetes is by far the commonest form of the disease, affecting 90–95 per cent of sufferers. In this type of diabetes the pancreas produces some insulin but not enough to fuel the body's cells – which may also become resistant to the little insulin there is. Many people with type-2 diabetes are completely unaware that they have the disease. It usually develops later in life, but it is becoming commoner in young people.

Type 2 is associated with obesity, poor eating habits and a modern sedentary lifestyle. The US Center for Disease Control and Prevention recently reported that the incidence of type-2 diabetes (sometimes known as adult-onset diabetes) has recently risen by 33 per cent, and about 16 million American adults currently have the condition. Complications related to diabetes are the sixth leading cause of death in the USA, and it is the leading cause of blindness in people aged between 20 and 70.

Hypothyroidism is a common cause of diabetes. Many complications of diabetes and hypothyroidism result from clogged arteries (see under **Cardiovascular disease (CVD)**, page 89).

What are the main symptoms?

Diabetics can have alternating periods of high or low blood-sugar levels. The symptoms of too much sugar in the blood include fatigue, extreme thirst, frequent urination, constantly feeling hungry, weight loss, eyesight problems and altered taste sensations – especially failure to identify that food is sweet. Symptoms of low blood-sugar levels include hunger, dizziness, sweating, confusion, palpitations and numbness or tingling of the lips. If low blood-sugar levels are not treated, further symptoms include double vision, trembling, disorientation, strange behaviour and, eventually, coma. The main danger with diabetes is from complications arising if insulin levels are not kept constant, which can cause the body to use its stored fat as fuel. When this happens, substances known as ketones can cause the body to become very acid. This is most common in type 1. Symptoms include nausea, difficulty in breathing, confusion progressing to coma, and breath that smells like nail-polish remover (acetone). People on high-protein, low-carbohydrate diets often have breath that smells like this too, reflecting their state of ketosis.

How is it diagnosed?

This usually involves analysis of sugar levels, initially in urine and subsequently in blood.

What is the conventional medical treatment?

Type-1 diabetes is usually treated by insulin injections. Type-2 diabetes is treated by diet and exercise, but oral or injected insulin may be necessary. Obesity is a major factor in this type of diabetes and significant weight loss is usually essential.

What are the foods involved?

We know many people who have controlled their type-2 diabetes by following our diet, bearing in mind the following specific factors.

It was once thought that people with diabetes should avoid sweetened food, and this is still important. However, eating some complex carbohydrates, especially refined products, can cause a greater rise in blood-sugar levels than sweet food. It is important, therefore, that people with diabetes should regulate their consumption of both simple and complex carbohydrates.

Our low-fat, high-fibre diet, which includes lots of raw vegetables and fruits as well as fresh vegetable juices, reduces the need for insulin and lowers levels of fat in the blood. The high fibre also helps to reduce surges in blood-sugar levels. Foods that are particularly helpful include:

- legumes, especially beans to help detoxify the pancreas;
- root vegetables;
- whole grains, but remember to regulate your intake of complex carbohydrates;
- foods that help to normalise blood-sugar levels, such as berries, fish, garlic, kelp, soya beans and most vegetables.

In addition, you should:

- keep saturated fats to a minimum;
- avoid all simple sugars, except when needed to correct blood-sugar levels;
- avoid salt and white-flour products;

- avoid man-made supplements such as large doses of vitamins – especially any containing the substance cysteine, which makes the absorption of insulin by cells worse;
- have black pepper and brewer's yeast, which are rich in chromium, helping glucose tolerance;
- eat regular meals;
- avoid special diabetic products, which can contain man-made sugars such as aspartame.

Choose from the list, on pages 48–71, of vegetables, fruit, herbs and spices that control blood-sugar levels, help regulate insulin or improve glucose tolerance.

DIGESTIVE-TRACT DISORDERS:
stomach and duodenal ulcers; small intestine (coeliac disease); Crohn's disease; large intestine (constipation, haemorrhoids and varicose veins; diverticulitis); irritable bowel syndrome

The digestive system (Figure 5), at its simplest, is a tube running from the mouth to the anus, which is designed to enable nutrients from food and drink to reach the blood, which then carries them around the body to nourish it. Digestion involves a combination of mechanical and chemical enzymatic processes to break down the huge molecules in proteins, fats and carbohydrates in food into smaller molecules that can be absorbed by the bloodstream and used by the body.

Food, which generally comprises very large molecules, is broken down by a series of enzymes in the mouth, stomach and intestine into much smaller molecules that can be absorbed into the bloodstream and used by our cells. Carbohydrates are broken down by amylases in the saliva and pancreatic juices in the small intestine, in alkaline conditions. Proteins are originally denatured in the stomach by pepsin in the strongly acid conditions that are needed to break the bonds between the constituent amino acids; and are subsequently broken down further by trypsin and chymotrypsin in the intestine. Fats are broken down by lipases in the intestine. The resulting mixture of what should be simple sugars, amino acids and fatty acids is absorbed through the intestinal wall directly or (in the case of fats) indirectly into the bloodstream to supply cells with small, low-molecular-weight

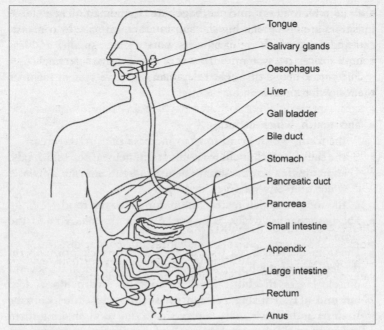

Figure 5 Digestive tract

substances that can be used to generate energy or synthesise protein, for example.

The number and type of teeth and the structure of our gut give us a good guide as to the diet that is best for us. Thus we have only four canine teeth for eating meat, and these are poorly developed. The remaining eight incisors and twenty molar and premolar teeth are best adapted to biting and grinding fruit, vegetables, grains, seeds and nuts. This is a good indication that we should not eat too much meat. The prevalence of dental caries in the West is a good indication that our diet contains far too much sugar. Tooth decay is very rare in rural areas of China and Japan, except where levels of fluorine in the environment are too high and people can lose most of their teeth.

Our digestive system is also that of an omnivore, in contrast with that of a herbivore or carnivore. The former have massive digestive systems – cows and sheep, for example, have a set of large stomachs that take up an enormous volume of their body and in which grass and herbage are fermented. Their large intestines are also much bigger than in other animals. In contrast, cats and dogs, which are carnivores, have a much smaller and less complex digestive system, with a very small 'large intestine'.

The path of food through the human digestive system includes the following organs and structures:

- The mouth, which includes:
  - the teeth, which grind food to increase the surface area;
  - the saliva, which includes a lubricant, neutralises acid foods, and contains antibacterial agents and the enzyme amylase, which converts starch to maltose;
  - the tongue, which tastes and manipulates the food.
- The oesophagus, which is the tube from the pharynx to the stomach.
- The stomach, which is a J-shaped expandable sack, normally on the left side of the upper abdomen, and which includes several muscle layers to churn food. It contains hydrochloric acid (around pH 2) strong enough to dissolve metal, which kills bacteria and helps denature proteins in our food, making them more vulnerable to attack by the enzyme pepsin, manufactured by the stomach. The stomach secretes mucus to protect itself from being digested by its own acid and enzymes.
- The small intestine, which has a length of about six metres and a large wrinkled and convoluted surface area for absorption: it also contains villi through which nutrients are absorbed. The total surface area is about 600m². Most enzymatic digestion occurs here. The secretions of the small intestine include amylase, maltase, sucrase and lactase to digest carbohydrates and lipase to digest fats. Several other associated organs secrete chemicals into the small intestine to aid digestion:
  - the pancreas secretes other enzymes and alkali solutions like bicarbonate as buffers;
  - the liver and gall bladder make and secrete bile, which contains salts to emulsify fat so it can be digested and increase pH to alkaline values (gallstones, normally composed mainly of cholesterol, can block bile ducts, causing pain and jaundice).
- The large intestine or colon, which begins with a lined pouch (which in humans is the appendix, a finger-like extension which

may play a role in the immune system). The large intestine's main function is to reabsorb water and to further absorb nutrients. It has a bacterial flora that includes *E. coli*, acidophilus bacteria and candida yeast, which produce gas as they ferment food. They also secrete beneficial chemicals such as vitamin K.

- The rectum, which is the last part of the large intestine. It stores faeces formed from digestive and other body wastes and opens to eliminate faeces at the anus.

STOMACH AND DUODENAL ULCERS

What is the disease?

Ulcers occur where the lining of the stomach or the beginning of the small intestine is eroded, leaving an internal open wound. They occur when the stomach or duodenum lining fails to provide adequate protection against the effects of digestive acid and enzymes. An ulcer is caused by the gastric secretions eating through the stomach (gastric or peptic ulcer) or intestinal (duodenal ulcer) wall.

Duodenal ulcers are caused by squirting of stomach acid into the first part of the small intestine, the duodenum.

What causes it and who does it affect?

Ulcers affect millions of people throughout the Western world every year, and it is estimated that they affect nearly 10 per cent of Americans at some point in their lives. It was once believed that stress and anxiety were the main causes. These may be contributory factors, but new evidence has shown that ulcers are often a result of an infection by a bacterium called *Helicobacter pylori*. These bacteria damage the mucus layer and lining of the digestive tract, and are thought to be transmitted from person to person. Some drugs, such as aspirin or other non-steroidal anti-inflammatory drugs, steroids, and other medication taken for arthritis can increase stomach acidity and lead to ulcers.

A common cause of ulcers is the consumption of over-the-counter antacids or calcium tablets. Consumption of antacids does just what their name suggests: they drastically change the pH of the stomach contents, interfering with pepsin's ability to digest protein. As the pH of the stomach rises above 4, the activity of pepsin decreases or stops. Some types of antacids made of sodium bicarbonate or calcium carbonate can be absorbed into the body, leading to kidney damage or other problems. Consuming antacids can actually increase the amount of acid secreted, as the stomach tries to restore its normal pH, and acid reflux may occur. So, use antacids only if prescribed by a doctor who has first carried out the simple breath test to diagnose *Helicobacter pylori* infection and reviewed your need for other medication that causes stomach acidity.

What are the main symptoms?

The symptoms of stomach ulcers include chronic burning or pain that begins up to an hour after eating or at night, and which is relieved by eating, vomiting or drinking a large glass of water. Other symptoms can include lower back pain, headaches, a choking sensation, nausea and vomiting.

How is it diagnosed?

The presence of an ulcer is diagnosed after drinking barium liquid followed by a series of X-rays of the stomach and duodenum or examination using a thin lighted tube attached to a camera inserted through the throat into the stomach and duodenum (endoscopy). The bacterial infection is usually diagnosed by a simple breath or blood test.

What is the conventional medical treatment?

Helicobacter pylori infection is treated with antibiotics. Otherwise treatment involves drugs or, in severe cases, surgery.

What are the foods involved?

The Plant Programme should help prevent and treat ulcers and the conditions that require the use of the medications such as aspirin that can cause them. The following are some of the key recommendations:

• Avoid all dairy produce, because the calcium and protein it contains stimulates the production of more acid; use soya, rice or other products instead.

- Avoid fried food, animal fats, black tea, coffee (including decaffeinated, which can be highly processed), chocolate, alcohol, carbonated drinks and soda water.
- Avoid added refined white sugar and salt totally.
- Eliminate refined carbohydrates.
- Eat foods high in vitamin E.
- Eat pineapple or papaya, to help with the digestion of protein.
- Flavour food with turmeric, which contains curcumin, which promotes healing.
- Eat alfalfa.
- Eat garlic, which is a selective antimicrobial, acting as a prebiotic for friendly bacteria.
- Eat plenty of dark-green leafy vegetables, which contain vitamin K needed for healing.
- If symptoms are severe, make a soothing dish by putting steamed vegetables through a blender or food mill.
- For rapid pain relief, drink a large glass of water with a little lemon juice added.

Other tips

- Take some essential fatty acids, such as evening primrose oil and fish oils.
- Buy acidophilus capsules – don't have yoghurt, but sprinkle the capsule contents on soya milk.
- Eat frequent small meals.
- Ensure that hot beverages have cooled before drinking them.
- Avoid tobacco smoke.
- Avoid the painkillers aspirin and ibuprofen.
- Avoid calcium and magnesium tablets. Try to eat foods that are rich in these minerals instead.

SMALL INTESTINE: COELIAC DISEASE

What is the disease?

Coeliac disease is a chronic digestive disorder. When a person with coeliac disease consumes gluten the small intestine swells and the tiny hairlike projections involved in absorbing vital nutrients from food are damaged and destroyed so that the person becomes undernourished; and frequently diarrhoea makes matters worse.

What causes it and who does it affect?

Coeliac disease is caused by a hereditary intolerance to gluten. Intolerance to other foods, especially lactose intolerance, may also occur, so avoiding dairy is a good idea. The disease affects both adults and children and can appear at any age, sometimes when a child is first introduced to cereal-based foods. It affects mostly Caucasians of European descent. Coeliac disease is much more prevalent than was once thought. As many as 1 in 500 people in North America and in Australia may be affected, with an even higher incidence in Western Europe.

> Don't give children under 6 months any of the gluten-containing cereals.

What are the main symptoms?

The first signs of coeliac disease are usually diarrhoea, weight loss and nutritional deficiency. Other symptoms can include nausea, anaemia, abdominal swelling, depression, fatigue, irritability, mouth ulcers, muscle cramps and wasting, and joint and/or bone pain. Infants may be small and below normal weight, with an anaemic, undernourished appearance. If left untreated, coeliac disease can be serious and even life-threatening, leading to many other disorders. For example, it can be a root cause of osteoporosis.

Coeliac disease is difficult to diagnose because the symptoms can be similar to those of other diseases such as irritable bowel syndrome and gastric ulcers. Because some people do not show clear symptoms, their condition may remain undiagnosed for a long time.

How is it diagnosed?

An accurate diagnosis requires a blood test, followed by a biopsy of intestinal tissue, usually a simple outpatient procedure. One doctor we know routinely screens all his patients for the condition and believes its incidence is much greater than acknowledged. Because the disease is hereditary, diagnosis in one family member should mean that all blood relatives are tested.

What is the conventional medical treatment?

There is no known cure, but the disease can be controlled effectively by strict adherence to a gluten-free diet and any damage to the gut can be completely reversed. Affected individuals generally return to normal health quickly after changing their diet, although older people may take longer to recover.

What are the foods involved?

Gluten is a general name given to the storage proteins (prolamins or gliadins), which are present in wheat, rye, barley and oats. The storage proteins of corn, rice and other good carbohydrates sources (see table below) do not contain these substances. Ideally, a gluten-free diet should contain no gluten ingredients, and all ingredients on food and drug labels should be carefully checked. 'Hidden' gluten can be an ingredient, especially in processed and fast foods such as prepared soups, salad dressings, sweets and desserts, and even some brands of soya sauce, tamari and rice syrups. Many additives, stabilisers and preservatives can contain gluten, so if in doubt check with the manufacturer. Moreover, some medications, toothpastes and mouthwashes can contain gluten, so always check with the pharmacist before buying such products.

Don't confuse the word 'glutinous' with gluten. Glutinous means gummy, sometimes used to describe rice and other 'sticky' foods because it reflects the type of starch a food contains, not its gluten content.

General guidelines for choosing gluten-free foods

The list in Table 6, on pages 108–109, is not comprehensive, and the Coeliac Society in the UK (www.coeliac.co.uk) publishes a list

Table 6 Foods for a gluten-free diet

Suitable foods	Unsuitable foods
Any rice including glutinous rice and rice products such as rice cakes and biscuits	Wheat (in general, the harder the wheat the higher its gluten content; durum wheat has a particularly high gluten content): • bulgar wheat, also sold as pilaf or tabbouleh • other wheat products, including farina, used to make hot cereals • orzo – rice-shaped pasta made from wheat • wheat flour Some soya sauces, including tamari
American corn (maize)	
Flours: • maize cornflour • cornmeal/polenta • potato flour • soya flour • arrowroot • lentil flour	Barley: • malt • malt vinegar • beer, ale, stout and lager • brown-rice syrup, often made with barley • yeast extract, including Marmite and Vegemite
Sago Tapioca	Rye and oats* and their products
Amaranth**	Triticale, a man-made cross between wheat (triticum) and rye (secale)
Flaxseed	Spelt, also known as German wheat
Quinoa** (which is very nutritious)	Semolina (made from large hard wheat grains retained after the hard flour has been removed)
Buckwheat** (which is botanically not a cereal)	Couscous (yellow granules of semolina from durum wheat)
Millet***, sorghum*** and wild rice***	Modified food starch or unidentified starch which may contain gluten
Cider or wine vinegar	Some dark vinegars
	Hydrolysed plant protein and hydrolysed vegetable protein, which may contain gluten

Table 6   *Continued*

Suitable foods	Unsuitable foods
	Some extracts and spices use starch fillers to improve the flow
Distilled alcoholic beverages, including gin, vodka, scotch whisky and rye whisky (distillation removes the prolamins)	
Wines and fortified wines	
	Some commercial thickened fruit-pie filling
	Canned or frozen vegetables in sauce
	Food thickened with flour, batter or crumbs, including processed meat, fish, sausages and pies
	Cereal-based coffee substitutes, malted cocoa beverages, barley water
	Custard powder, stock cubes and some baking powders
	Certain brands of baked beans
	Foods containing E953 or E965

*According to a review in the *Journal of the American Dietetic Association* in May 2001, 'current scientific evidence more strongly supports the conclusion that oats are safe than it does that oats are harmful'.
**These grains are only very distantly related to gluten-containing grains, but no clinical trials have been carried out to ensure that they are safe for people sensitive to gluten.
***Millet and sorghum are more closely related to maize than to wheat, and wild rice has a protein profile similar to cultivated rice, so these foods are considered to be safe.

With all the above foods, check for yourself if they cause you symptoms.

of gluten-free manufactured products in a booklet that is updated every year. Some manufacturers use a gluten-free symbol on their labels. A wide range of specially manufactured foods such as bread, pasta, biscuits and cake can be prescribed in the UK by the NHS.

Note: even 'allowed' grains can be contaminated with gluten-containing grains during harvest, transport, milling and/or processing.

Other helpful dietary advice includes:

- Take acidophilus bacteria (but not in dairy yoghurt). Buy capsules, remove the contents from the gelatine capsules and add to soya milk or soya yoghurt.
- Ensure a good intake of iron by including small quantities of eggs or meat, pulses, lentils, nuts and green vegetables daily.
- Sip fruit juice or herbal or green tea rather than coffee with meals.

CROHN'S DISEASE

What is the disease?

Crohn's disease is an inflammatory bowel disease. It usually affects the lower part of the small intestine, but can affect any other part of the digestive tract. Left untreated, it can become an extremely serious condition.

What causes it and who does it affect?

It has been suggested by some that it is caused by a bacterium that survives the pasteurisation of milk. Milk is an excellent cultural medium for the growth and transmission of many unpleasant bacteria and micro-organisms. A bacterium called *Mycobacterium paratuberculosis* causes chronic enteritis in cows, known as Johne's disease, which is an incurable chronic infectious disease characterised by diarrhoea, weight loss and debility. It is one of the most widespread bacterial diseases of domestic animals throughout the world and of cows in the UK. It has been suggested that it can cause Crohn's disease in humans. Recent research at Liverpool University has confirmed this link.

Crohn's disease is thought to affect a relatively small number of people and affects men and women of all ages equally. Children with the disease may suffer delayed development and stunted growth because of nutritional deficiencies.

What are the main symptoms?

The disease causes inflammation that extends deep into the lining of the intestine, causing cramping abdominal pain, diarrhoea, bleeding from the rectum, loss of appetite and weight loss. The intestine can become blocked by scar tissue and the disease can also cause sores or ulcers. People with the disease commonly suffer from nutritional deficiencies. The onset can be associated with alarming symptoms such as high fever, weight loss of more than two kilos in a few days, severe abdominal pain and rectal bleeding. If the disease continues for many years it can become extremely serious.

How is it diagnosed?

It is difficult to diagnose because its symptoms are similar to other diseases of the intestines, especially ulcerative colitis. It can appear intermittently. Blood tests are used to check for anaemia and high white-blood-cell count; X-rays are used to look at the small intestine, and a long flexible lighted tube linked to a computer may be used to examine the lining of the small intestine (endoscopy).

What is the conventional medical treatment?

According to orthodox medicine, there is no known cure. The treatment is aimed at controlling inflammation, often involving the use of steroids, relieving symptoms and correcting nutritional deficiencies. The use of steroids can, in turn, lead to osteoporosis in the long term.

What are the foods involved?

Our first advice is to give up all dairy produce, since milk may carry the bacterium responsible for the disease. Another reason to give up dairy food is that it is high in histamine and it also contains carrageenan, which is used to stabilise milk proteins and has been shown to cause intestinal problems in laboratory animals.

In addition, we advise you to:

- Maintain a diet that includes lots of fresh cooked vegetables.
- Avoid fried and greasy food.
- Avoid processed meat and pickles, alcohol, caffeine, fizzy drinks and any foods with artificial additives and preservatives.
- Avoid refined sugar and artificial sweeteners.
- Drink lots of liquids, such as high-quality water (see page 46), herbal teas and fresh juices.

Two close friends who had been diagnosed with the disease and who have kept to the Plant Programme have been symptomless from the time Jane discovered the suggested link between Johne's disease in cows and Crohn's disease in humans.

LARGE INTESTINE: CONSTIPATION, HAEMORRHOIDS AND VARICOSE VEINS

What is the disease?

The above large intestine disorders are characterised by a difficulty in passing stools, or the irregular passage of hard dry stools as a result of food moving slowly through the large intestine.

What causes it and who does it affect?

Most people have constipation from time to time in their life. It is almost always due to a bad diet lacking in fibre and fluids, and is particularly common in those following a high-protein low-carbohydrate diet. It may be a side effect of taking iron supplements (especially during pregnancy), painkillers, antidepressants and several other medications.

What are the main symptoms?

Some doctors think it is acceptable to go to the toilet three times a week, while others maintain it is essential to have a bowel movement at least once a day. We agree with the latter advice.

Constipation can give rise to bad breath, flatulence, obesity and malabsorption. Few people realise its association with piles (haemorrhoids) and varicose veins, when the presence of large stools causes the bowel to sag and prevents the flow of blood back to the heart from the veins around the anus or the legs.

What is the conventional medical treatment?

Usually laxatives, but stimulant laxatives that irritate the bowel walls can cause damage leading to dependency on the laxative. The fact that doctors prescribe laxatives, some of which can cause serious side effects, instead of recommending safe natural products is a serious concern.

What are the foods involved?

We do not think that anyone following the Plant Programme diet will suffer from this condition. Giving up cheese, alone, should help greatly. See also the diet for Crohn's disease and remember that beans, prunes, figs, pears, dried apricots and linseed are among the best natural laxatives.

LARGE INTESTINE: DIVERTICULITIS

What is the disease?

It is a condition in which small saclike protrusions form in the wall of the large intestine.

What causes it and who does it affect?

Diverticulitis typically occurs in people consuming a low-fibre diet, leading to stools that are hard and difficult to pass and that require increased pressure to force them through the bowel. Once the protrusions develop they do not go away, but they may not cause symptoms if they do not become inflamed. If, however, they do become infected or inflamed they can cause fever, chills, nausea and pain. The disease can be acute (sharp, intense) or chronic (of long duration).

The condition affects older rather than younger people, usually from the age of about fifty onwards, because the walls of the intestine weaken with age. It is thought to affect many millions of people in the West, who often attribute their symptoms to indigestion. Diverticulitis mainly affects people with poor eating habits, a family history of the disease, and obesity.

What are the main symptoms?

Cramping, flatulence, constipation or diarrhoea, and an almost continual need to go to the toilet. There may be blood in the stool. Peritonitis can develop if the intestine ruptures.

How is it diagnosed?

Liquid barium, which is opaque to X-rays, is passed into the colon using an enema, and X-rays are then used to show up abnormalities in the intestine. Also, a thin flexible lighted tube can be inserted into the rectum to examine the lower colon and, if necessary, remove tissue samples for examination.

What is the conventional medical treatment?

Dietary changes and, if that fails, surgery in extreme cases. Antibiotics are used if the diverticula are infected.

What are the foods involved?

The key is to consume an adequate amount of fibre (at least 30g per day) and lots of quality water (at least eight glasses or about two litres per day). Linseed is particularly good for this condition. Eat protein from vegetable sources and fish, with lots of well-cooked brown rice, plenty of leafy green vegetables and a great deal of garlic. Totally eliminate dairy products, red meat, refined sugar and its products, and fried and processed food. In acute attacks you may be advised to go on a low-fibre diet – eat steamed vegetables only. Always take high-fibre foods, such as cereals, separately because they can bind zinc, iron and other essential nutrients so they cannot be absorbed.

IRRITABLE BOWEL SYNDROME (IBS)

What is the disease?

In IBS the contractions of the digestive tract become uncoordinated, interfering with the normal passage of food and waste through the intestine. This sets up a partial obstruction, trapping gas and stools and causing distension and constipation. It is painful but generally not serious.

What causes it and who does it affect?

The cause of the condition is unknown, although some scientists believe a virus or bacterium may play a role (see also under Crohn's disease). It is the commonest digestive disorder in the West, affecting about one in five Americans. It affects twice as many women as men, and the age of onset is usually between 25 and 45.

What are the main symptoms?

There are no physical signs of the disease in bowel tissue. Symptoms may include abdominal pain, constipation often alternating with diarrhoea, flatulence, mucus in the stools, and nausea – and sometimes severe headaches and vomiting. The condition is often associated with malnutrition. Some patients with IBS also have arthritis of the ankles, knees and wrists.

How is it diagnosed?

The first step is to rule out disorders with similar symptoms such as coeliac disease, tumours, Crohn's disease, depression, diverticulitis, infectious diarrhoea, ulcerative colitis and lactose intolerance. The following procedures may be used to do this: barium enema, endoscopy, rectal biopsy, and stool examination to check for the presence of blood, bacteria and/or parasites.

What is the conventional medical treatment?

Most people are advised to increase the amount of protein in the diet, take mineral and vitamin supplements, and exercise regularly.

What are the foods involved?

Although the condition is less serious than diverticulitis, a similar diet is appropriate.

EATING DISORDERS:
obesity, anorexia, bulimia

Adult animals tend to maintain a relatively constant weight, known as their set weight, which is regulated on a timescale of weeks or longer. Hence, if an animal is starved and then allowed access to food it will eat much more food than normally. Conversely, if an animal is force-fed and then allowed access to food it will not eat very much. Interestingly, when food is restricted, the base metabolic rate decreases, which is one reason why it is so difficult to lose weight by dieting based on restricting food intake: it is better to change the type of food you eat by following the Plant Programme.

In this section we discuss extreme eating disorders, from obesity to anorexia. Our diet will simply help you to have the weight and body shape that is right for you. It will not give you a tall, slim, leggy figure if you are naturally small and short-waisted, as we are! No diet will.

OBESITY

What is the disease?

An excess of body fat is usually defined as more than 20 per cent higher than ideal body weight, as calculated for age, gender, build and height. In healthy women, 25 per cent of the body weight can be fat and in healthy men 17 per cent. Obesity contributes directly to cardiovascular disease by increasing blood pressure, cholesterol and triglyceride levels. It is also associated with high blood-sugar levels and diabetes incidence, which also predisposes to cardiovascular disease and many other illnesses.

What causes it and who does it affect?

Most of the extra calories we eat but do not need immediately are stored in fat cells, a survival mechanism from our early ancestors to provide a food store for times when no food was available. Instead of being a valuable survival mechanism, the body's ability to store fat is now more likely to damage health. Even moderate obesity puts stress on the back, legs and internal organs. It increases the body's resistance to insulin and its susceptibility to infection, increases the risk of coronary artery disease, increases blood pressure and the risk of stroke and insulin-resistant or type-2 diabetes as well as the risk of several types of cancer. It is also a factor in gall-bladder and kidney disease. More than half of all American adults are overweight, and the proportion of people in many Western countries, including Britain, is fast reaching a similar level. An increasing number of children and teenagers are obese, putting them at risk of heart attack, stroke, colon cancer or gout, regardless of whether they slim down in later life. One theory is that obesity is caused by eating too much refined food: these foods lack essential nutrients, leaving the body unsatisfied and hungry for more food, thereby setting up a vicious circle of cravings. This helps to explain why high-protein diets, which supply minerals, may be so popular among people trying to lose weight.

Other causes include glandular problems (especially of the thyroid), diabetes, hypoglycaemia, anaemia and food intolerances.

Obesity may be associated with a dependence on over-sweetened foods. Many people feel the need to eat something sweet after a meal, but this is a habit that can be broken.

What are the main symptoms?

Too much body fat.

How is it diagnosed?

It is formally diagnosed by calculating the body mass index (BMI) from a combination of weight and height. Charts to calculate your BMI are available (on the Internet, for example), but the recommendations do vary between one chart and another and they do not take account of differences in build. Being 'apple-shaped', with waist measurement exceeding hip measurement, is a simple indication, but we recommend you request help from your health professional rather than trying to self-diagnose your condition.

What is the conventional medical treatment?

Appetite-suppressing drugs, exercise and, in extreme cases, people may have their jaw clamped or their stomach operated on to reduce absorption. Doctors rarely have time to supervise diet, which essentially means eating better food with fewer calories.

What are the foods involved?

One of the key issues is eating over-refined foods so that the body continues to crave nutrients that have been taken out. Eating fatty foods is also a key factor, especially saturated fats or oils hydrogenated to make margarine, which can contain high levels of trans-fatty acids. The human taste for fatty foods has been considered to be a survival mechanism from our ancestors who needed to store energy. Calories from fat are more easily converted to body fat than calories from other sources.

- Don't count calories; just eat good food by following the principles of the Plant Programme and using the recipes in our books. These recommend lots of complex carbohydrates, but this does not mean bland, tasteless meals. Our recipes are delicious, practical and easy to make, as well as being healthy and nutritious.
- Eat balanced meals consisting of small amounts of animal protein, larger quantities of vegetable protein (such as soya, lentils and other pulses, cereals and nuts), small amounts of good fats (such as extra-virgin cold-pressed oils) and complex carbohydrates.
- Never drink commercial fizzy drinks – and that includes those described as diet drinks. Drink sparkling water mixed with fruit juice instead, or herbal and green teas with a slice of lemon. One study found that using artificial sweeteners increased weight gain because they increased appetite and slowed down digestion.
- Eat lots of fresh raw or lightly cooked fruit and vegetables – if cooked they should be lightly steamed, baked, grilled or stir-fried, using only good unrefined vegetable oils.
- Fennel is a natural appetite suppressant.
- Turmeric improves digestion, increases energy and helps to remove fat from the blood.
- Onions and garlic contain natural detergents that help to move fat from the liver.
- Avoid anything that contains refined sugar, as this triggers the release of insulin, which promotes the storage of fat in the body.
- Limit alcohol consumption.

Other tips

- Keep a diet diary to help you keep an accurate record of what you are eating.
- Always grill rather than fry food.
- Always eat breakfast, even if it is just a piece of fruit.
- Don't skip meals; make your main meal lunch, not dinner.
- Avoid crash dieting, which can cause your metabolism to slow down. In particular, avoid fad diets, which can produce spectacular weight loss over the short term but can be very unhealthy (see page 10). Also, once you stop such diets the weight often returns.
- Observe the conventional advice to take plenty of exercise.

ANOREXIA NERVOSA AND BULIMIA NERVOSA

What is the disease?

The name anorexia nervosa is used to describe people who, although thin and weak, continue to try to lose weight, in some cases eating too little food to stay alive. Other symptoms include intense fear of becoming fat no matter how thin the person becomes, extreme hyperactivity, an obsession with exercising and negative feelings about body image.

Many people who are anorexic are also bulimics. Bulimics binge on large quantities of food – usually high-calorie food – quickly and then make themselves vomit. They may also use laxatives or enemas or other ways of purging the body, usually in secret. Unlike people with anorexia, whose self-starvation becomes obvious, bulimics can hide their problems, sometimes for years, because many maintain their weight in the normal range.

What causes it and who does it affect?

The cause is not fully understood and is suspected by some doctors to have a psychological basis, perhaps reflecting an imbalance of the neurotransmitter serotonin in the brain. Some anorexia sufferers have been found to have severe zinc deficiency, but it is not clear if this is a cause or a symptom. Most sufferers of both illnesses are female and the conditions typically appear during adolescence, although they can affect women up to the age of forty and older. The incidence has escalated dramatically during recent years and as many as one person in fifty may be affected at some time in their life in parts of the Western world. Some people with anorexia struggle with the condition all their life, while others can outgrow it – though where people have had the acute phase of the disorder, serious long-term damage to the body may have been caused.

What are the main symptoms?

Some people with anorexia just stop eating, or make themselves vomit immediately after eating, some take laxatives, and some do all three. Most people with anorexia have trained themselves to ignore normal feelings of hunger. They may spend hours, however, reading recipes and even preparing elegant meals for others. They deny there is anything wrong with them and usually say they are simply not hungry.

One of the main symptoms of bulimics is trips to the bathroom after meals and the sudden disappearance of large quantities of food.

Anorexia and bulimia can lead to extreme weakness, dizziness, irregular periods or complete cessation of menstruation, osteoporosis, ulcers, hair loss, erosion of tooth enamel from repeated vomiting, broken blood vessels in the face, and low pulse rate and blood pressure. Other physiological changes include thyroid and other glandular problems, irregular heartbeat and, in serious cases, heart failure and death.

How is it diagnosed?

From the symptoms above and based on a detailed case history. Dentists frequently diagnose bulimia by observing that teeth have been eroded by regurgitated stomach acid.

What is the conventional medical treatment?

Conventionally it is treated by fortified milk-based drinks containing a complete range of nutrients including zinc. Antidepressants may also be prescribed. Psychotherapy and counselling may be helpful.

What are the foods involved?

We have found that people with this condition want to be in control, and following the Plant Programme closely has helped some young women that we know to do this, with a great improvement to their health and wellbeing. One highly intelligent young woman, badly affected by anorexia as well as appalling acne, recovered in weeks after changing from her milk-based drink diet to our programme.

The following guidelines are particularly important:

- Eliminate foods likely to cause allergies or intolerance, such as dairy and wheat.
- Avoid all sugar, junk food and refined white flour.
- Eat a high-fibre diet with as many vegetable proteins and complex carbohydrates as possible.
- Eat smaller, more frequent portions and ensure that you have breakfast.
- Buy a variety of healthy snacks such as nuts, seeds and dried and fresh fruit, and leave them around to nibble when you can.
- Chew your food slowly and well.
- Drink lots of fresh water and herbal teas.

MENOPAUSAL SYMPTOMS

What is the disease?

This is not a disease but a natural progression, similar to puberty. It is the point at which a woman stops ovulating and menstruating, signalling an end of fertility.

What causes it and who does it affect?

It normally occurs around the age of 47 in Europe, but it can be much earlier.

Smokers, and those with chronic eating disorders or who have had certain cancer treatment, can be at particular risk of early menopause. Many years before a woman stops ovulating, the production of the hormones oestrogen, progesterone and testosterone slows down. Oestrogen and progesterone are both reproductive hormones, and oestrogen also affects the functioning of many other organs and systems in the body, including the breasts, bladder, skin, bones, cardiovascular system, liver and brain. Although oestrogen levels drop sharply after menopause, other organs take over from the ovaries and continue to produce a less potent form of the hormone. Progesterone also has effects beyond the reproductive system, including on the brain and nervous system, while a woman's testosterone level is most important for sex drive.

What are the main symptoms?

Women's experiences vary greatly. Some experience minimal symptoms or none at all. In others, symptoms can include some or all of the following: anxiety, skin problems (especially dry skin), fatigue, bloating, headaches, heart palpitations, hot flushes (especially night sweats), insomnia, irritability, decreased sex drive, poor concentration, mood swings, urinary incontinence, vaginal drying and itching, and weight gain. After menopause, most women are at increased risk of CVD and osteoporosis.

Many of the symptoms ascribed to menopause can be caused by poor thyroid function (see page 143).

How is it diagnosed?

Usually a case history and in some cases blood tests to determine circulating levels of hormones.

What is the conventional medical treatment?

Initially, the simplistic view was that most menopausal symptoms are caused by loss of oestrogen, so the treatment was simply to replace this with oestrogen replacement therapy (ORT, or ERT in North America). It soon became apparent that prescribing unopposed oestrogen increased the risk of endometrial cancer. The treatment was therefore replaced with oestrogen combined with man-made progesterone called progestin (hormone replacement therapy – HRT), which some studies have shown to increase the risk of breast cancer, coronary heart disease and strokes.

What are the foods involved?

Our diet, which includes many foods containing lots of natural phyto-oestrogens and phytoprogesterone, has limited our own symptoms. Japanese women generally experience far fewer symptoms than Western women, and this is attributed to the higher content of phyto-oestrogens in their diet. We both use cream containing wild yam. Black cohosh and red clover are herbs traditionally taken by Chinese and Western women, respectively, to counteract menopausal symptoms. The authoritative *The Desktop Guide to Complementary and Alternative Medicine* indicates that there are no known contra-indications for phyto-oestrogens consumed as part of diet, although there are concerns about taking concentrated supplements. The guide concludes that increasing consumption of phyto-oestrogens in the diet has few risks and various potential health benefits.

Our diet contains high levels of these protective substances, and many women report a great improvement in their symptoms. We suggest that you ensure you have plenty of the following:

- soya milk – at least one glass every day
- tofu and/or miso
- unrefined whole-grain cereal, especially flaxseeds
- pulses such as beans, peas or lentils
- lots of fruit, especially berries, pomegranates and dates
- vegetables, especially fennel and sprouting seeds such as alfalfa
- lots of filtered boiled water
- herbs, especially anise, red clover and sage
- herb teas, especially camomile, sage and valerian

In addition, make sure that your diet contains 50 per cent raw uncooked foods, you consume only minimal amounts of coffee, chocolate and other substances high in caffeine, and that you keep alcohol intake to moderate levels.

MULTIPLE SCLEROSIS

What is the disease?

Multiple sclerosis (MS), also known as disseminated sclerosis, is an autoimmune condition in which the immune system attacks the central nervous system, leading to demyelination of nerves in the white matter of the brain and spinal cord. The name 'multiple sclerosis' refers to the scars (scleroses) in the white matter, which is mainly composed of myelin. Myelin is a fatty substance that insulates nerves so they can transmit electrical signals. Hence demyelination damages the ability of nerve cells to communicate with each other.

Life expectancy of patients is nearly the same as that of the unaffected population.

What causes it and who does it affect?

Much is known about the disease processes involved in MS, but according to most medical texts the cause remains unknown. As with other autoimmune diseases, however, the immune system attacks tissues (in this case the nervous system), probably as a result of exposure to a molecule that has a similar structure to one of its own. Theories include genetics or infections, and/or environmental factors. As discussed on page 84, there is strong circumstantial evidence of a link with the consumption of dairy products, and there is also evidence that even in high-risk countries those who have oily fish as their main source of animal protein are at lower risk.

Individual attacks can be triggered by infections such as the common cold, influenza, gastroenteritis or stress.

MS has a prevalence of between 2 per 100,000 at low latitudes and 150 per 100,000 at high latitudes (up to 200 in 100,000 in northern Scandinavia). It has been suggested that vitamin D deficiency due to lack of sunlight could explain this latitude gradient, but dairy consumption has been shown to be a more likely explanation. A dietary link is supported by several migration studies, which show that if migration occurs before the age of fifteen, the migrant acquires the new region's susceptibility to MS, whereas if migration occurs after fifteen, the migrant retains the susceptibility of their home country. The Canary Islands, for example, where there is a large expatriate European population, have a much higher incidence of MS than would be predicted by their latitude.

Chemicals called dithiocarbamates, which are used as fungicides in agriculture and in the rubber industry are associated with demyelination in laboratory animals, and some arsenic compounds can also cause demyelination.

MS usually appears in adults in their thirties, but it can also appear in children. The primary progressive subtype is more common in people in their fifties. As with many autoimmune disorders, the disease is more common in women, although in people over fifty, MS affects males and females almost equally.

What are the main symptons?

Symptoms can include changes in sensation, muscle weakness, spasms, difficulty in moving, lack of co-ordination and balance, problems with speech or swallowing, visual problems, fatigue, acute or chronic pain, and bladder and bowel difficulties. Cognitive difficulties can occur, together with symptoms of depression or unstable mood. The main clinical measure of disability progression and symptom severity is the Expanded Disability Status Scale (EDSS).

Symptoms may seem worse if the temperature is high.

How is it diagnosed?

Symptoms alone may be sufficient for a diagnosis of MS. However, the condition is often difficult to diagnose, since symptoms may be similar to other conditions and it is necessary to rule these out. Simple tests which involve measuring reactions to optical or sensory stimuli may be used. Otherwise, magnetic resonance imaging (MRI) can be used to identify areas of demyelination, and a lumbar puncture may be carried out to look for evidence of chronic inflammation of the central nervous system.

What is the conventional medical treatment?

There is no known cure for MS. Treatments attempt to return function after an attack, prevent new attacks and prevent disability, usually using immunosuppressant drugs such as steroids. Orthodox medications used to treat MS can have unpleasant side effects, and many patients pursue alternative treatments, including the use of cannabis. The prognosis is difficult to predict;

it depends on the type of the disease, the individual patient's disease characteristics, the initial symptoms and the degree of disability the person experiences as time advances. The latest research into stem-cell treatment suggests that this may help to arrest the course of the disease and in some cases reverse it. Even so, we think you should consider changing your diet.

What are the foods involved?

- On the precautionary principle, all dairy produce should be avoided.
- Meat eating may be a factor, if protein molecules similar to those in myelin are ingested. Oily fish appears to be protective.
- A diet that contains vegetable protein and fish as the main source of dietary protein is likely to be most beneficial.
- Intake of saturated and trans-fats should be low, with higher levels of polyunsaturated (see page 38) from vegetable sources and oily fish.
- Eating organically produced food helps to reduce exposure to pesticides, many of which are neurotoxic and some of which have been shown to cause demyelination in experimental animals.

MYALGIC ENCEPHALOPATHY (ME), CHRONIC FATIGUE SYNDROME (CFS)

What is the disease?

Myalgic encephalopathy (ME), also known (particularly in America) as chronic fatigue syndrome (CFS) is associated with extreme physical and mental tiredness (fatigue), which seriously interferes with a person's daily life and has lasted for more than six months. Even normal physical activity can make sufferers very tired. ME/CFS is not infectious although some people develop it after an infection; glandular fever and some flu strains are thought to be common triggers for the condition. Many people who develop ME/CFS were previously fit and active.

The condition has been known since the 1930s among doctors of many countries, but between 1970 and recently it was often dismissed as being all in the mind – as reflected by its nickname 'yuppie flu' – despite the fact that patients who develop ME/CFS were typically functioning at a high level before being affected by illness. The condition is now recognised by the World Health Organisation and the UK Department of Health as a real, long-term disease.

What causes it and who does it affect?

There are several theories to explain ME/CFS, for example that it is linked to depression or disorders of the immune system or the hormonal system. Some research indicates that the nervous system is also involved in ME/CFS. Other suggested triggers for the condition have included viruses (including chronic Epstein Barr virus infection), Lyme disease, total allergy syndrome, multiple chemical sensitivity syndrome and chronic systemic candidiasis.

The best scientific evidence links the condition to problems with the mitochondria, the organelles in cells responsible for oxidising food such as glucose to generate energy via the citric acid (Krebs) cycle. If this cycle is impaired, energy generation in the body is inadequate, leading to chronic fatigue and the generation of toxic chemicals instead of the substances needed by the body. For example, large quantities of lactic acid (which normally limit athletes' performance) can be generated after minimal exercise in those with ME/CFS. Tartaric acid, which is a toxin that affects mood, muscles and kidney function, is frequently high in the urine of patients with ME/CFS (and fibromyalgia). Problems with the Krebs cycle can be initiated by infection, by taking antibiotics (mitochondria have many affinities with bacteria) or by taking certain recreational drugs (especially if they are contaminated with damaging chemicals). Other chemicals in the environment, such as antiseptics designed to target bacteria, could be involved although there is no scientific evidence for this. Some pesticides, including phenylamide, fungicides and the insecticides rotenone (which is broad spectrum) and diafenthiuran (which is used against mites) interfere with the Krebs cycle.

Mitochondrial impairment can lead to problems with heart function (which explains why patients feel much better lying down); this, in turn, can affect other organs.

ME/CFS can affect anyone. The precise number of people with the condition is not known. Studies from a broad variety of countries, including the USA, UK and Australia, have produced a wide range of findings. For instance, in the USA, it has been suggested that the condition affects at least four to ten adults out of every 100,000 over the age of eighteen. In the UK, a Royal Colleges' report estimated that the illness was much more common, affecting 1–2 per cent of the population. A study in Australia found thirty-seven cases per 100,000 people. Some of these figures may well be underestimates.

ME/CFS can affect any age group, but most commonly starts in people aged between the early twenties and mid forties. In children, the most common age of onset is thirteen to fifteen, but it can occur in children as young as five. The endemic form is commoner in women, but in epidemics it is equally common in men and women. It is also more likely to be diagnosed in white (non-Hispanic) people than in other ethnic groups.

What are the main symptoms?

Common symptoms include: muscle and joint pain in the absence of swelling; fatigue that lasts more than twenty-four hours after previously normal levels of exercise; forgetfulness, memory loss, confusion or difficulty concentrating; sleep disturbances; and/or flu-like symptoms. Other symptoms can include: palpitations; sweating; feeling faint or having problems with balance; painful glands in the neck or armpits; a sore throat; headaches; feeling sick; and mood swings. The severity of symptoms can vary from day to day. If you suffer from such symptoms you should consult your doctor.

Studies have shown that patients with ME/CFS have a disproportionate incidence of psychiatric conditions such as anxiety disorders and depression. This may reflect the production of neurotoxic chemicals by a malfunctioning Krebs cycle, just as a malfunctioning boiler in your house emits toxins. Another factor of course is that people who suffer from any long-term conditions that seriously interfere with their lives, such as cancer, MS or AIDS, are liable to suffer from depression or anxiety as a response to their condition.

For some sufferers, ME/CFS is lifelong, but nowadays most patients can recover within two years especially if they are given good science-based advice.

How is it diagnosed?

Your doctor will normally take a case history and carry out a physical examination. Most doctors regard ME/CFS as a difficult condition to diagnose because there are usually no physical symptoms; for example, joint pain is not accompanied by swelling. Blood tests are usually performed to rule out other illnesses, but most doctors are presently unaware of the biochemical tests that are available specifically for ME/CFS.

What is the conventional medical treatment?

The usual treatment for ME/CFS aims to manage symptoms and may involve graded exercise therapy (it is worth remembering that too much exercise can send patients to bed for weeks or months), learning to pace yourself in your day-to-day activities and cognitive behavioural therapy, together with pain relief based on drugs such as ibuprofen or paracetamol for muscle and joint pain, headaches and other physical symptoms. Sufferers may also be prescribed tricyclic antidepressants. Complementary treatments such as relaxation therapy, acupuncture or homeopathy may be recommended.

Some doctors prescribe antibiotics and antiviral drugs (including doxycycline, amantadine and acyclovir), medications that affect the immune system, steroids (including the synthetic steroid fludrocortisone, alone or in combination with the beta-blocker drug atenolol), cimetidine or ranitidine (antihistamines used to treat heartburn) to treat the symptoms of ME/CFS. Sleeping pills may be prescribed for sleep disturbance.

What needs to be done?

For the best diagnosis and treatment, the results of appropriate biochemical tests should be used to correct problems with a defective Krebs cycle. The problem is that the treatments vary greatly from person to person depending on which part of the complex Krebs cycle is affected. Treatment normally involves simple minerals, vitamin compounds or simple sugars, so there is not much profit to be made by the pharmaceutical companies. There is therefore little marketing or publicity to inform doctors.

Unfortunately, sufferers are usually persuaded to adapt and cope with ME/CFS for months and sometimes years instead of being properly diagnosed and treated following precise biochemical tests.

If children with ME/CFS are unable to attend school, it is important to consult the local ME/CFS association at an early stage.

What are the foods involved?

We emphasise that blood tests should be carried out to identify the precise chemical problems with the Krebs cycle in patients and the appropriate supplements prescribed. (In case of difficulty please visit www.janeplant.com and write to info@janeplant.com.)

- We also recommend that you give up foods that could contain antibiotic residues, such as dairy produce and industrially produced meat. Eat small amounts of animal protein such as organically produced free-range eggs, wild fish (taking care to avoid oily fish such as salmon, which contain concentrations of pollutants; take ultrapure cod-liver oil instead) or wild meat such as venison or rabbit.
- Eat a highly alkaline diet to help neutralise the lactic acid that can be produced in large quantities by a malfunctioning Krebs cycle and which is often responsible for symptoms such as joint pain. We recommend a diet with a ratio of 80:20 per cent alkalising to acidifying foods. See the chart on page 28–29.
- Eat organically produced fruit and vegetables, herbs and spices to ensure good nutrients, while avoiding pesticides that could aggravate symptoms.
- Take a B-complex vitamin supplement (including vitamin B12) and foods that are good sources of B vitamins (see page 48–71).
- Take a magnesium gluconate supplement if blood tests show a deficiency in magnesium.
- Foods containing tartaric acid must be avoided. These include anything with baker's yeast. It is also available as a food additive in baking powder, grape- and lime-flavoured beverages, and poultry. It may also be found in grapes and grape products, including wine. Cream of tartar, which may be used for baking, is nearly pure tartaric acid. It is a common food additive, E472.

- Many people also recommend a gluten-free diet, and there is comprehensive information on this under **Coeliac disease** on page 105.

SKELETAL DISORDERS:
Osteoarthritis and rheumatoid arthritis, osteoporosis

The human skeleton is a unique structure that is important in defining our species. It comprises more than 200 bones, each of which has a distinct shape that reflects its function. It is important to realise that our bones are living, growing tissues – like the liver, lungs, or any other organ in the body. Bone, like all human tissue, is made of various types of cells, well supplied with blood vessels and with nerves and pain receptors.

The skeleton has several distinct functions. It is the principal structural support for the muscles, enabling us to stand upright and move about. It is also protective against both outside forces and those generated by our own muscles. Movement of the bones is controlled by muscles, as instructed by the brain. The skeleton is also the body's main store of calcium and other alkali metals and bases, which the body can release to neutralise the blood if it becomes too acid, as is likely on the typical Western diet.

OSTEOARTHRITIS AND RHEUMATOID ARTHRITIS

What are the diseases?

In healthy joints, adjoining movable bones are covered with a layer of cartilage surrounded by a fluid-filled capsule of tough fibrous tissue (ligaments). The viscous fluid is secreted into the joint by a thin (synovial) membrane. Arthritis can result from problems with the synovial membrane, secretions of synovial fluid, or damage to bone, cartilage or ligaments. The two commonest forms of arthritis are osteoarthritis and rheumatoid arthritis.

Osteoarthritis involves deterioration of the cartilage protecting the ends of bones, which, in severe cases, can break down so that the normally smooth sliding surfaces of the joint become rough.

Rheumatoid arthritis is considered to be an autoimmune or 'self-attacking-self' disease, whereby the synovial membrane and cartilage and tissues in and around the joints and bone surfaces are damaged. The damaged tissue is replaced with scar tissue in severe cases eventually causing bones to fuse together.

What causes it and who does it affect?

Arthritis can be caused by viral, bacterial or fungal infections. Osteoarthritis, according to conventional medicine, mostly reflects wear and tear of joints with ageing, and it is generally considered to be a disease of old age. It affects more men than women. On the other hand, rheumatoid arthritis frequently occurs in people under forty years of age, mostly females, and can affect children under the age of sixteen. Unlike osteoarthritis, which affects individual joints, rheumatoid arthritis can affect all the synovial joints (see also under **Autoimmune diseases**, page 84). Arthritis and other diseases of the skeleton and muscles are the primary source of disability in many Western countries.

What are the symptoms?

Arthritis is inflammation of one or more joints and is associated with pain and stiffness, especially in the mornings, a diminished range of movement and, in severe cases, swelling and deformity with bone spurs developing in affected joints.

Osteoarthritis most often affects the knees, hips and back but also commonly attacks the hands and knuckles. Eventually any affected joints can become deformed, painful and stiff.

Rheumatoid arthritis causes stiffness, swelling, fatigue, anaemia, weight loss, fever and, often, severe pain.

Lyme disease is caused by a tick-borne bacterium and has symptoms that mimic arthritis. This disease can be diagnosed using blood samples.

How is it diagnosed?

Physical examination, blood tests and scanning.

What is the conventional medical treatment?

Osteoarthritis may be treated initially with aspirin and other non-steroidal anti-inflammatory drugs (NSAIDs), but since these tend to generate acid they may not help in the long term. Pharmaceutical aspirin and the other NSAIDs can produce an acid reaction, causing stomach problems. In advanced cases of osteo-arthritis of joints, replacement surgery may be required.

One anti-inflammatory drug that is sometimes prescribed for both osteo- and rheumatoid arthritis works by inhibiting an enzyme that causes inflammation, without causing the stomach problems associated with taking NSAIDs. A relatively new drug used to treat rheumatoid arthritis blocks the action of a protein, called tumour necrosis factor, which is normally involved in fighting infection. In some people the use of this drug has led to increased susceptibility to serious infection. Cortisone treatment may be used for rheumatoid arthritis.

What are the foods involved?

Both osteo- and rheumatoid arthritis can be helped greatly and in some cases reversed with proper diet and lifestyle changes.

In the case of osteoarthritis make sure the ratio of acid to alkaline foods in the diet is balanced, with a ratio of 60:40 of alkali-generating to acid-generating food for prevention and 80:20 for treatment of these conditions, using the table on pages 28–29.

Particularly helpful foods include:

- ginger, alfalfa, hot peppers (cayenne pepper and chilli), nettle-leaf tea and celery, but be sure to have natural products not extracts;
- eggs, asparagus, garlic and onions, which contain sulphur, which is needed to maintain the skeleton;
- turmeric, which contains curcumin and is commonly used in curry powder, and has both anti-inflammatory and pain-relieving properties;
- sea cucumber, which is a rich source of lubricating compounds for joints and joint fluid (available in some Asian shops);
- garlic, which has powerful antibacterial, antiviral and anti-fungal properties;
- fresh pineapple, which contains an enzyme that helps to reduce inflammation;
- oily fish and fish oils, but buy only brands (e.g. Seven Seas ultra-pure variety) that are treated to ensure that they contain

levels of toxic pollutants such as PCBs and dioxins that are as low as possible.

Check the list on pages 43–71 for vegetables, fruits, herbs and spices that are rich in anti-inflammatory compounds or natural aspirin.
Avoid:

- any products containing man-made fluoride, including tooth-paste and mouthwash;
- iron supplements and multivitamin tablets containing iron.

Some distinguished doctors treat rheumatoid arthritis as food intolerance. See further under **Allergies and intolerances to food** (page 72).

Other tips

- Take aspirin, but in its natural form as wintergreen. It is an alcohol and was modified by Bayer to prepare pharmaceutical aspirin, which can produce an acid reaction in the body. Wintergreen is available from all good herbalists.
- Chrondroitin sulphate and glucosamine sulphate are two supplements that people with osteoarthritis find helpful.
- Take kelp, which is rich in minerals that maintain skeletal health.
- Rheumatoid arthritis may be helped by taking evening primrose oil.

OSTEOPOROSIS

What is the disease?

Osteoporosis (the word means porous bones) is a disease charac-terised by low bone mass, leading to fragile bones and increased risk of fracture – particularly of the hips, spine and wrist. In advanced cases there may be a massive change of posture (dowager's hump) and height.

What causes it and who does it affect?

Bone is constantly being remodelled by cells called osteoclasts, which break down old bone, and osteoblasts, which build up new bone under the influence of hormones and bone-generating growth factors. In osteoporotic bone, fewer osteoblasts are available, or their activity is impaired. In advanced osteoporosis, bone is poorly mineralised and its organic matrix may degenerate. The conventional wisdom is that bone is at its strongest at around the age of thirty and that it begins to decline thereafter, with a dramatic fall in women after the menopause. The disease is suggested to reflect failure to accumulate adequate bone mass until early adulthood or to too rapid a loss in later life.

One in three women and one in twelve men over the age of fifty suffer from osteoporosis in the UK. In the USA, it is predicted that one in two women and one in eight men over the age of fifty will have an osteoporosis-related fracture at some time. Although osteoporosis can affect young people with eating disorders or on some types of medication, it is mainly a disease of older women. Women are generally more affected, because of their hormonal and physiological make-up. Both sexes can also suffer from bone loss as a side effect of medications including anti-convulsant, chemotherapeutic and corticosteroid drugs, and thyroid hormone treatment. Aromatase inhibitors, used against breast cancer, can affect bone density. Aluminium antacids, including those that are self-prescribed, can also cause a decrease in bone mass. There is some suggestion that osteoporosis may have a hereditary component.

Many people, including health professionals, attribute osteoporosis almost entirely to dietary calcium deficiency, which they say can be remedied by taking calcium supplements or eating dairy produce. There is much evidence against this, however, in that Western countries with high dairy consumption, where calcium deficiency is highly unlikely, have an incidence of hip fracture in women over fifty that is up to two hundred times that of Nigeria and China, which traditionally consume low-dairy diets. The World Health Organisation (WHO) confirms that countries with relatively low intakes of calcium do not have an increased incidence of osteoporosis. Indeed, they note that dietary calcium levels similar to those proposed to prevent osteoporosis can cause several adverse biological effects. It is now thought that for the vast majority of people the answer to osteoporosis does not lie in boosting calcium intake but in limiting calcium loss.

This involves reducing the amount of acid in the body caused by a diet high in animal proteins such as hard cheese and processed meat (see Table 2).

What are the main symptoms?

Osteoporosis has been called the 'silent disease' because it may be symptomless until there is a fracture. Fractures of the hip and wrist are particularly common.

How is it diagnosed?

It is normally diagnosed by bone-density measurement. The most commonly used techniques include dual-energy X-ray absorptiometry (DEXA or DXA) or dual-photon absorptiometry (DPA), whereby the loss of beam energy is used to calculate bone mineral density. The result is calculated by computer and compared with a WHO standard to give a risk of fracture.

What is the conventional medical treatment?

Calcium supplements, with or without vitamin D, are used for both prevention and treatment, although they can have unwanted side effects, including gastrointestinal upsets and depression, fatigue and kidney problems, respectively. In the case of menopausal women, hormone replacement therapy may be prescribed, although this has been shown to increase the risk of breast cancer, heart disease and stroke. Bisphosphonates, which work by damaging osteoclasts, may be prescribed, although they can cause gastrointestinal upsets. The hormone calcitonin can be given by injection, but this can cause nausea, vomiting and facial flushing.

What are the foods involved?

The latest research underlines the importance of balancing acid-generating and alkali-generating foods in the diet so that excess acid generated by a typical Western diet, high in cheese, meat and refined carbohydrates, does not leach calcium from the bones. Use the table on pages 28–29 to help you to achieve a balance of 60 per cent alkali-generating foods (herbs, spices, fruit and vegetables) to 40 per cent acid-generating foods, to protect against developing osteoporosis, or a balance of 80 to 20 if you already have the disease. In addition:

- Good sources of calcium include most dark-green vegetables, fish with bones, hazelnuts, kelp and other sea vegetables, molasses, oats, sesame seeds and spread (tahini), tofu and wheat germ.
- Magnesium helps to promote bone growth, and a deficiency can affect the production of vitamin D, leading to osteoporosis. Magnesium is a constituent of chlorophyll and is abundant in green vegetables. Other sources include whole grains, wheat germ, molasses, seeds and nuts, apples and figs.
- Garlic, onions and eggs contain sulphur, which is needed for healthy bones.
- Soya and other substances rich in phyto-oestrogens help to substitute for the body's loss of oestrogen after the menopause.
- Caffeine, alcohol and many drugs appear to cause a loss of bone density. A study of women aged 36 to 45 found that those who drank two cups of coffee per day suffered a net calcium loss of 22mg per day.
- Limit alcohol intake, because there is some evidence that it interferes with calcium absorption.
- Avoid sugar, salt and other substances containing sodium, which can increase calcium excretion (see page 41).

Other tips

- Sunlight helps your skin to produce vitamin D, which is essential for the proper absorption of calcium.
- Weight-bearing exercise is important for bone mineralisation.
- Avoid smoking, which increases the body burden of cadmium, which damages bone.
- Avoid fluoride, including in toothpaste and mouthwashes, which causes pathological change in bone.
- Avoid aluminium (found in some antacids), tin and endocrine-disrupting chemicals, which can affect oestrogen metabolism.
- See also our book *Osteoporosis: Understanding, Preventing and Overcoming*.

SKIN PROBLEMS:
acne, dermatitis, eczema, psoriasis

The skin is the largest organ of the body. It is covered by an oil-and-water emulsion and consists of three layers, the epidermis (or outer layer), the dermis (middle layer) and the subcutaneous layer, which is often fatty. The skin eliminates a significant proportion of the body's toxic waste products. If the body contains more toxins than the kidneys and liver can eliminate, the skin takes over. This is a key factor behind many skin disorders, including acne.

The skin also protects the body and helps maintain shape. It provides a first line of defence against infection, parasites and pollution. The natural layer of oil-and-water emulsion is the first barrier against invasion by bacteria, fungi and yeast. The outer layer of the skin, the epidermis, contains white cells, which kill bacteria, and other special cells that remove pollutants to lymph glands and in some cases are responsible for allergic skin conditions.

The skin helps to lower body temperature when it is hot, by perspiration, while the fat layer of the skin helps to prevent heat loss when it is cold, by absorbing warm infrared rays. Heat control in the skin is also maintained by the dilation and contraction of blood vessels.

ACNE

What is the disease?

Acne is an inflammatory skin disease characterised by pimples, blackheads and white-heads. It causes much emotional distress, which can lead to psychological problems.

What causes it and who does it affect?

It often arises first during teenage years and is regarded by most orthodox doctors as a side effect of the production of male sex hormones in both girls and boys. These hormones are thought to stimulate the production of a type of protein and an oily substance called sebum. Blemishes are thought to arise if sebum is secreted faster than it can be removed through the pores, the excess oil encouraging the growth of bacteria. Blackheads form when pores become blocked, when sebum combines with skin pigments. White-heads form when this happens below the surface of the skin. Contrary to common belief, acne is not caused by a lack of cleanliness.

Other factors thought to contribute to acne include heredity, oily skin, hormonal imbalance, allergies, stress and the use of certain drugs such as steroids, lithium, oral contraceptives and some epileptic drugs, pollution and a body pH that is too acidic. Nutritionally, it has been linked to a diet high in saturated and trans-fatty acids and other animal products. Our experience and communications from readers suggest that it can be eliminated by following the Plant Programme – and especially by eliminating all dairy products and refined carbohydrate foods.

Acne may develop because of the fat content in dairy foods. Hormones and steroids that modern dairy and other animal products often contain upset the body's natural hormone balance.

Acne affects 80 per cent of all Americans between the ages of 12 and 44 and has become the most commonly treated skin condition in the USA. Although onset frequently occurs at puberty, it is increasingly affecting adults.

What are the main symptoms?

Pimples, blackheads and white-heads, some of which become infected and can leave the skin permanently scarred.

How is it diagnosed?

Visual examination.

What is the conventional medical treatment?

Antibiotics, antiseptic skin creams and, in some cases, hormone treatment.

What are the foods involved?

Keep closely to the Plant Programme, and especially avoid:

• dairy produce, including milk, cream, butter, yoghurt and cheese, and animal meats, especially cheap minced beef; these are commonly found in favourite teenage foods such as burgers (plain or with cheese), pizzas, ice cream and milk chocolate;

- refined carbohydrates, including white sugar, white bread and, again, pizza bases and burgers;
- milk with tea or coffee;
- animal fats, such as lard;
- too many eggs.

And ensure you have:

- a high-fibre diet, with lots of vegetables, nuts and fruit;
- foods rich in zinc, including soya beans, whole grains, and sunflower and pumpkin seeds;
- foods rich in vitamins A, C and E, including fruit, vegetables and whole-grain cereals;
- lots of water and freshly made juices.

DERMATITIS AND ECZEMA (see also under **Allergies and intolerances to food**, page 72)

What is the disease?

Dermatitis is a general term for any type of inflammation of the skin. Often the term dermatitis is used interchangeably with eczema, though strictly the latter term refers specifically to atopic dermatitis which is associated with scaling, flaking, thickening, weeping and often severe itching of the skin.

What causes it and who does it affect?

Stress, especially chronic stress, can cause or exacerbate all forms of dermatitis. Atopic dermatitis, or atopic eczema, which typically appears on the face, the bends of the elbows and behind the knees, generally affects allergy-prone individuals during the first five years of life. Other forms of dermatitis and eczema are linked to the consumption of dairy products and/or gluten. Many cases are simply the result of allergies to substances such as nickel (in jewellery, for example) that the skin is in contact with, but this is beyond the scope of this book. Underlying problems include food intolerances and allergies.

What are the main symptoms?

Itchy, sore lesions on the skin or scalp.

How is it diagnosed?

Visual examination and case history.

What is the conventional medical treatment?

Steroid creams, but if used for too long they can thin the skin.

What are the foods involved?

The condition of virtually all skin disorders improves if dairy products and foods containing gluten are eliminated from the diet. Other allergies and intolerances to food should also be considered (see page 72). The following supplements may be helpful:

- Brewer's yeast, because it contains B vitamins and minerals such as zinc, which are needed for a healthy skin
- Kelp, which contains minerals that help skin healing
- Foods high in vitamins C and E
- Essential fatty acids, including evening primrose and fish oils
- Camomile tea, which can help reduce inflammation

See the list on pages 48–71 for vegetables, fruits, herbs and spices that contain anti-inflammatory agents.

Other tips

- Tea-tree oil can be helpful, applied to the affected skin.
- Limit the number of baths, since these destroy the skin's protective emulsion.
- Avoid the use of bubble bath, shower gel, and similar toiletries.
- Use simple, unperfumed soap, or simply clean affected areas with olive oil; bath water can be softened by adding simple, unperfumed bath salts.
- Use cotton bedding and clothing, and ensure that detergents are thoroughly rinsed out after washing.
- Avoid the use of household chemicals, especially air fresheners and any perfumed bathroom, kitchen or polish sprays.
- Never wear perfume, including perfumed cosmetics and deodorants.

PSORIASIS

What is the disease?

The condition is caused by the rapid growth of the skin's outer layer of cells, which fail to mature, and appear as scaly patches that can spread to cover larger and larger areas. Despite its appearance, the condition is not contagious.

What causes it and who does it affect?

It most commonly begins between the ages of 15 and 25. The underlying cause is not known, but it is commonest in countries following a Western diet. Attacks are thought to be triggered by stress and general debility, including following viral or bacterial infection, and can also be triggered by the use of some drugs, including NSAIDs (used for treatment of arthritic conditions), lithium (used for bipolar depression) and beta-blockers (for heart disease and high blood pressure). People with HIV/AIDS often have psoriasis.

What are the main symptoms?

Reddish-brown patches of skin covered with silvery-white scales, usually on the legs, knees, arms, elbows, scalp and ears. The toenails and fingernails of sufferers can appear ridged and pitted. Some people have associated arthritis that is similar to rheumatoid arthritis and difficult to treat.

How is it diagnosed?

Visual examination and case history.

What is the conventional medical treatment?

There is no known cure. Conventional treatment is aimed at treating the symptoms using ointments to soften the scales. Sometimes ultraviolet light is used, combined with tar or with other drugs to remove itchy scales and skin debris. Cortisone cream is often prescribed, but long-term use can thin the skin. Some types of vitamin D ointment may also provide symptomatic relief. Some drugs taken orally are also used, but they can have potentially serious side effects, so ensure that you discuss them with your doctor.

What are the foods involved?

- Follow our diet by eating at least 50 per cent of raw vegetables and fruits or their juices; include grains and a little fatty fish in the diet as well.
- Eat plenty of dietary fibre (see under **Irritable bowel syndrome**, page 114).
- Consume fish oil, flaxseed oil and evening primrose oil, which help to prevent the inflammatory response.
- Avoid all red meat and dairy products, which promote inflammation.
- Do not consume any fried foods, processed foods, saturated fats, sugar or refined white flour.
- Follow our advice on the right balance of omega-3 and omega-6 fatty acids (see Food Factor 6).

THYROID PROBLEMS:
hyperthyroidism, hypothyroidism

The thyroid gland is the biggest gland in the neck. It is shaped like a butterfly, with two wings or lobes wrapped around the trachea or windpipe at the front of the neck. The only known function of the thyroid is to make hormones that affect nearly all tissues in the body by increasing cellular activity, so it is important in regulating the body's metabolism. The thyroid gland can be affected by several problems, some of which are extremely common. These include the production of too much or too little hormone (hyperthyroidism and hypothyroidism respectively), goitre (sometimes associated with the production of too much thyroid hormone, but normally reflecting enlargement of the thyroid gland because it is not producing enough thyroid hormone), inflammation of the thyroid, the formation of nodules or lumps in the gland, and cancer. Here we are concerned mainly with hyperthyroidism and hypothyroidism, but the advice should be useful in maintaining thyroid health generally. Hyperthyroidism is not as common as hypothyroidism. Both disorders affect more women than men. Many endocrine-disrupting chemicals, for example BHC (used in pesticides), PCBs (remaining in the environment following their use in the electronics industry in the 1970s) and polybrominated flame retardants (used to fireproof furnishings) can all affect thyroid-hormone function.

HYPERTHYROIDISM

What is the disease?

In those with a healthy thyroid, just the right amounts of two hormones, T4 and T3, are produced. These regulate the metabolism, affecting how many calories we burn, how warm we feel, and how much we weigh. These hormones also affect most other organs: for example, the heart beats harder and faster under the influence of thyroid hormones. Hyperthyroidism is caused by overproduction of thyroid hormones.

What causes it and who does it affect?

There are several causes of the condition. Usually the whole gland is overproducing thyroid hormones, although in some cases excess hormone production may be caused by a single nodule. One of the commonest causes is Graves' disease, named after the Irish doctor who first described it, which is thought to be an autoimmune disease whereby the patient's immune system attacks the thyroid gland. In addition to hyperthyroidism, this is associated with inflammation and swelling of the tissues around the eyes and thickening of the skin over the lower legs. Graves' disease affects about eight times more women than men. It is more common in thirty- to forty-year-olds and tends to run in families. Thyroiditis, thought to be caused by a virus, can also lead to the release of excessive amounts of thyroid hormones. Hyperthyroidism can also occur in patients whose doses of thyroid-hormone medication are too high, particularly that containing T3, which is needed in only small amounts.

What are the main symptoms?

Although there are several different causes of this condition, most of the symptoms are the same and typically include a constant

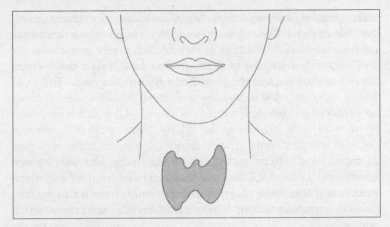

Figure 7   Thyroid gland

feeling of being hot, increased perspiration, nervousness, depression, irritability, insomnia and fatigue, increased bowel movement, less frequent menstruation with decreased menstrual flow, hair and weight loss, separation of nails from the nail bed, trembling hands, rapid and sometimes irregular heartbeat (palpitations) and in some cases protruding eyeballs. Sometimes the onset of symptoms is so gradual that it may be months before people realise they are ill. Thyroiditis (inflammation of the thyroid) causes the typical symptoms of hyperthyroidism, but they generally last for only a few weeks.

How is it diagnosed?

Normally a firm diagnosis requires blood tests to determine the levels of circulating thyroid hormones.

What is the conventional medical treatment?

Temporary forms of hyperthyroidism caused by thyroiditis or excessive thyroid medication may be treated with beta-blockers to improve symptoms such as hand-shaking or palpitations. For patients with chronic hyperthyroidism, caused by Graves' disease or a type of goitre, anti-thyroid medications are used to suppress thyroid-hormone production. These can have side effects such as rashes, itching or fever and (rarely) can produce liver inflammation, associated with yellowing of the skin, or deficiency in white blood cells, accompanied by a high fever and/or a severe sore throat.

A major shortcoming of these medications is that their effects are not permanent and the condition often comes back. The most widely recommended permanent treatment involves administering an oral dose of radioactive iodine (iodine-131), which is absorbed by thyroid cells, damaging or killing them. Because iodine is concentrated primarily in the thyroid, there is little radiation damage or side effects to the rest of the body. The only known adverse side effect is if too many thyroid cells are killed by the treatment. More rarely, surgery may be used to remove part of the thyroid, especially where hyperthyroidism is caused by a single nodule.

What are the foods involved?

In addition to the general principles of the Plant Programme, the following foods, which contain goitrogenic substances, can help to suppress the production of thyroid hormones: broccoli, Brussels sprouts, cabbage, cassava, cauliflower, kale, mustard greens, peaches, pears, rutabagas, rape seed and rape-seed oil, soya beans, spinach and turnips. The goitrogens are often damaged by cooking, so eat the vegetables raw or very lightly cooked – or drink juices. Except in serious cases it may be worth trying these dietary changes before rushing into surgery or treatment with radioactive iodine. Large amounts of vitamins and minerals are needed for this hypermetabolic condition, so follow the Plant Programme carefully. Because man-made endocrine-disrupting chemicals can affect thyroid function, it is particularly important to pay attention to Food Factor 1, which is aimed at reducing exposure to harmful chemicals.

Other tips

- Brewer's yeast may be helpful, because it is rich in basic nutrients including the B vitamins needed for thyroid function.
- Kelp and seaweed may also be helpful as a source of iodine and other minerals, while the lecithin in soya helps to protect the lining of cells, which can be damaged in this condition.

- Do not take vitamin E tablets or capsules, because these can further stimulate the thyroid gland.

HYPOTHYROIDISM

What is the disease?

Hypothyroidism is caused by underproduction of thyroid hormones.

What causes it and who does it affect?

Hypothyroidism affects about 15 million people in the USA, and affects nine times as many women as men, usually between the ages of thirty and fifty. Millions of people throughout the West are thought to have hypothyroidism that is undiagnosed. It can also be caused by an autoimmune condition called Hashimoto's disease, which is accompanied by goitre. In this condition, inflammation of the thyroid gland can kill or damage a large percentage of thyroid cells. This disease can be associated with pernicious anaemia, lupus (an autoimmune disease), yeast infections and rheumatoid arthritis. Hypothyroidism can also be caused by radioactive iodine treatment or surgery, or, in rare cases, because levels of thyroid-stimulating hormone (TSH), which is produced by the body's master gland, the pituitary, and helps regulate thyroid-hormone production, are too low. The disease can also be caused by poor diet, which is lacking iodine, selenium and/or cobalt, with too high levels of goitrogenic substances, excessive fluoride, excessive consumption of unsaturated fats or pesticide residues, ionising radiation, alcohol and some drugs, including narcotics and sedatives.

What are the main symptoms?

The commonest symptoms are fatigue and an inability to tolerate cold. Other symptoms include loss of appetite accompanied by weight gain, a slow heart rate, painful premenstrual periods, muscle cramp and weakness, dry, rough skin, hair loss, recurrent infections, migraine, hoarseness, constipation, depression, goitre and drooping swollen eyes. Some patients might have only one of these symptoms, while others will have combinations.

How is it diagnosed?

It is diagnosed by measuring levels of thyroid hormones in the blood and by measuring levels of TSH. TSH levels are generally high in hypothyroidism as a result of the pituitary trying to stimulate the thyroid to produce more hormone. An iodine absorption test using a small amount of radioactive iodine may be performed to reveal a low uptake of iodine, indicative of hypothyroidism. In some patients, more detailed tests carried out by an endocrinologist may be needed.

What is the conventional medical treatment?

It is normally treated with thyroid hormone tablets, which must be taken for life. The important thing is to identify the correct dose.

What are the foods involved?

Kelp and other marine food substances that are enriched in iodine, the essential component of thyroid hormone, are particularly helpful. Taking this, combined with strictly limiting the amounts of raw or lightly cooked goitrogenic foods (see under 'Hyperthyroidism', above) in the diet can improve this condition dramatically. We have helped several friends and colleagues to improve this condition with just this simple advice, and one friend found that her large goitre stopped growing. It is unfortunate that doctors generally do not give out this simple advice. Apricots, dates, molasses, prunes, raw seeds and whole grains are also beneficial.

Other tips

- Brewer's yeast contains many mineral nutrients as well as B vitamins which are also essential for thyroid function.
- Avoid taking sulphur drugs or antihistamines, fluoride and chlorine, which block iodine receptors in the thyroid gland.

URINARY-TRACT DISORDERS:
kidney disease, kidney stones, urinary-tract infections

The kidneys remove waste products of metabolism from the body, keep chemicals in balance, including, importantly, pH, and help to maintain the body's water balance. The waste fluid, or urine, passes from the kidneys into two tubes called the ureters, which pass into the bladder. This acts as a temporary store for urine before it is excreted through the urethra. There are several different conditions that may affect the kidneys.

KIDNEY DISEASE (RENAL FAILURE)

What is the disease?

Inflammation of the kidney, caused by any of a wide range of conditions, leading in serious cases to kidney failure.

What causes it and who does it affect?

The kidneys may be damaged by exposure to some drugs, including chemotherapeutic agents and high doses of the painkiller ibuprofen, as well as environmental pollutants including heavy metals (especially cadmium and lead) and pesticides. Renal failure can also result from many other disorders, including congestive heart failure, chronic hypertension, diabetes and liver disease. Infectious illnesses, such as measles, scarlet fever and tonsillitis, can also cause kidney damage. Cystitis, which is not itself a serious health problem, can lead to kidney infection if it is left untreated.

Bright's disease of the kidneys is associated with the presence of blood in the urine, high blood pressure and water retention (oedema). Inflammation of the tiny blood vessels that filter out waste from the blood may occur as a result of an immune response, for example to streptococcal throat infection. The kidney and the structure into which urine is discharged from the kidney (the renal pelvis) may become filled with urine because of an obstruction. Polycystic kidney disease, whereby cysts render the kidneys incapable of functioning, is an inherited condition. In renal tubular acidosis, bicarbonate is not reabsorbed normally, causing impaired acid excretion, which can lead to severe acidosis, potassium depletion and bone disorders.

What are the main symptoms?

One of the most important symptoms of kidney disease is fluid retention, which is associated with limited urine production and accumulation of salt and other waste in the body. The ankles and hands may swell and the patient is likely to be short of breath. Toxic waste may accumulate in the bloodstream. Other symptoms of kidney disease include abdominal and/or back pain (which can be sudden and intense), chills, fever, loss of appetite, nausea and vomiting, and urinary urgency. The urine may be cloudy, foul smelling and/or bloody.

How is it diagnosed?

Urine samples are tested for levels of albumin, waste products from metabolism in muscle cells, haemoglobin, phosphorus, potassium and urea. Special X-rays performed after injecting iodine (which is opaque to X-rays) may be used, as well as modern scanning methods.

What is the conventional medical treatment?

In severe cases of kidney failure, dialysis may be required, and even kidney transplantation.

What are the foods involved?

To prevent and treat kidney disease, drink lots of fluid, especially filtered boiled water. Also:

- Consume a diet high in raw food, that includes asparagus, bananas, celery, cucumber, garlic, papaya, parsley, potatoes, pulses, seeds (especially pumpkin seeds), sprouting seeds, watercress and watermelon.
- Eliminate salt and potassium chloride (a salt substitute).
- Avoid animal protein foods such as eggs, meat, fish and dairy produce, because this can exacerbate kidney disease and lead to the accumulation of protein in the kidney, which makes matters worse. The best protein sources include pulses such as beans (including adzuki and kidney beans), lentils, peas and soya products, and whole grains.
- Drink plenty of vegetable and fruit juices.

Other tips

- Brewer's yeast contains important mineral nutrients and B vitamins, helps kidney function and reduces fluid retention.

- Lecithin contained in soya helps to treat kidney inflammation or nephritis.
- Spirulina (a plant plankton) may also help to reduce kidney disease if it is caused by mercury and drugs.

KIDNEY STONES

What is the disease?

Kidney stones (renal calculi) are accumulations of minerals that lodge in the urinary tract.

What causes it and who does it affect?

Human urine is often almost saturated with uric acid, phosphate and oxalate. Normally pH control and the presence of other chemicals mean that these substances remain in solution. In some cases, however, crystals may begin to form, which can aggregate into stones large enough to restrict urinary flow. Dehydration can be a factor in the formation of kidney stones, because urine becomes more concentrated, increasing the likelihood of precipitation.

There are four kinds of kidney stones: calcium oxalate (the commonest), uric acid stones, magnesium ammonium phosphate (struvite) stones and cystine stones.

- Calcium oxalate stones reflect high circulating levels of calcium, which can result from disease of the tiny glands in the neck that regulate blood calcium levels, or from vitamin D poisoning. A diet too high in animal protein is also liable to generate too much acidity and lead to this condition. Consumption of refined sugar, which can cause high levels of circulating insulin, can, in turn, increase the amounts of calcium to be excreted in the urine.
- Uric acid stones form when urine is particularly concentrated and/or blood levels of uric acid are high, a condition associated with gout.
- Struvite stones are caused by infection and are commonest in women who suffer from recurrent urinary-tract infections.
- Cysteine stones are caused by a rare congenital defect.

About one person in ten in Western countries is estimated to have kidney stones at some time in their life. They are rare in childhood, but can occur in the twenties and are commonest in white men aged between thirty and sixty. Kidney stones are ten times more common now than at the start of the twentieth century. Calcium oxalate stones often run in families, and can affect people with Crohn's disease or irritable bowel syndrome.

What are the main symptoms?

Symptoms include back pain, radiating from the upper back to the kidney area just above the waist, profuse sweating, frequent urination, pus and blood in the urine, odorous or cloudy urine, absence of urine formation, and sometimes chills and fever. This can be one of the most painful of all health disorders. In less severe cases, symptoms may resemble gastroenteritis.

How is it diagnosed?

In acute cases, kidney stones are diagnosed on the basis of the symptoms presented. They are also diagnosed using a special method of X-ray whereby iodine, which is opaque to X-rays, is injected; as it is excreted, it can be used to show the structure of the kidney. Other types of scans can also be used.

What is the conventional medical treatment?

In some cases, drinking large quantities of pure water, combined with effective pain relief, may allow small kidney stones to pass naturally. Alternatively, ultrasound may be used to break up the stones into smaller fragments (lithotripsy), which can then be flushed out with urine. In some cases an operation may be necessary.

What are the foods involved?

General guidelines for preventing and treating kidney stones include the following:

- Drink plenty of high-quality water. This is the most important way to prevent kidney stones. For pain relief, fresh lemon juice diluted in water at frequent intervals can help.

- Avoid salt or potassium chloride (salt substitute) and fizzy drinks.
- Do not omit calcium-containing foods from the diet – but we do not recommend taking calcium supplements.

Dietary changes can help to control the development of kidney stones. The diet depends on the type of stone: refer to the table on pages 28–29, which lists foods that are acid-generating and those that are alkali-generating. For calcium oxalate stones, it is considered helpful to make the urine more alkaline. Therefore, the recommended high fluid intake should be achieved by drinking alkalising (i.e. alkali-rich, phosphorus-poor) beverages such as green tea, wine, beer (in moderation) and fruit and vegetable juices. Also, minimise your consumption of animal protein and increase the proportion of vegetables, fruit, herbs and spices in your diet. A diet high in animal protein, especially cheese and processed meat, produces excessive amounts of acid in the body, which causes the body to excrete calcium.

- Do drink fresh fruit juice, especially of citrus fruit (lemon, lime, orange, grapefruit).
- Magnesium increases the solubility of calcium oxalate, reducing the risk of stone formation. Good sources include seafood, brown rice and soya products such as tofu.
- Orange-coloured fruit and vegetables, rich in vitamin A, such as apricots, cantaloupes, carrots, pumpkins and sweet potatoes help to prevent kidney-stone formation.

But:

- Do not drink coffee, because it contains relatively high amounts of oxalate, and excess intake increases renal calcium loss.

For struvite or calcium phosphate stones, both of which are poorly soluble in alkaline urine, solubility can be increased and precipitation inhibited by acidification of urine. For patients with uric acid stones, urine should be adjusted to a slightly acid value. Acidification of the urine is best achieved by increasing the proportion of vegetable protein, such as pulses, cereals and other seeds, and nuts, relative to fruit, vegetables, herbs and spices.

We do not all digest and metabolise foods in the same way. Your individual metabolism may determine whether a food leaves an acid or alkaline residue in the body. For example, certain foods containing organic acids, such as citrus fruits and tomatoes, which normally leave no acid residues, may be incompletely metabolised in some people and are thus acid-forming for them. This may occur where stomach acid is low or thyroid activity is subnormal.

URINARY-TRACT INFECTIONS (UTIs)

What is the disease?

UTIs include infections of the kidneys, bladder or urethra, the first of these being the least common. They normally involve bacteria, usually found in the intestine, although chlamydia (a sexually transmitted organism) may also be responsible for infection.

What causes it and who does it affect?

Both men and women suffer from UTIs, including those of the bladder. Urethritis (infection of the urethra), cystitis (infection of the bladder) and pyelonephritis (kidney infection) are more common in women, especially during pregnancy. This is because of the close proximity of the anus, vagina and urethra and the short length of the urethra in females, which facilitates transmission of bacteria from the anus to the bladder via the urethra, which can occur during sexual intercourse. UTIs in men may indicate serious underlying conditions such as diseases of the prostate gland or bladder cancer. Urethritis in men is most often contracted sexually. UTIs may also affect those with diabetes and multiple sclerosis.

Shrinking of the urethral and vaginal membranes after the menopause can increase the risk of bladder infections.

In some cases, inflammation of the bladder can be unrelated to infection. It can be caused by chemotherapeutic and other drugs, too much alcohol, or other irritants including food allergies or other food intolerances.

What are the main symptoms?

Bladder infections are characterised by urgency to urinate, which is typically frequent and painful. The urine may appear cloudy and have a strong, unpleasant smell, and there may be blood in the urine.

How is it diagnosed?

A doctor may use paper indicators to dip into urine samples to confirm the presence of albumin, white blood cells or blood in the urine. Ideally, samples will be tested to identify the organism involved. The presence of white blood cells and/or blood in the urine does not necessarily indicate infection, especially if samples are clear and smell normal.

What is the conventional medical treatment?

Antibiotics are generally used, and potassium citrate is given to relieve pain and discomfort. Before taking antibiotics, you should ensure that a urine sample is tested to identify the specific organism involved; this may be difficult after antibiotics have been used. Try to limit the use of antibiotics, because they can promote the development of antibiotic-resistant strains of bacteria, requiring the use of even more powerful antibiotics, with the risk of increased side effects.

Where the cystitis is related to irritation rather than infection, antibiotics should be avoided and the condition treated by drinking lots of still (not fizzy), high-quality water.

What are the foods involved?

- In the case of infections and irritation, you should drink plenty of high-quality still water, with regular drinks of unsweetened cranberry juice for infections.
- Celery, parsley and watermelon, and their juices, act as natural diuretics and cleansers.
- Fresh blueberry is particularly helpful in UTIs, because of the activity of substances contained in the blue pigment.
- Avoid alcohol, caffeine, carbonated beverages, coffee, chocolate, all refined and processed food, sugar and sugary foods.
- Avoid taking zinc or iron supplements, which can encourage bacterial growth.

Other tips

- Make sure that you drink adequate amounts of fluid and urinate regularly.
- Women should ensure that they sit upright when urinating, to ensure that the bladder empties completely.
- It is important to keep the genital and anal areas clean and dry.
- Women should wipe from front to back after emptying the bladder or bowels.
- Wear underwear made of cotton, not man-made fibres.
- Never use commercial feminine hygiene sprays, douches, bubble baths, sanitary ware or toilet paper that are perfumed, since the chemicals used can cause irritation.
- Plain unperfumed soap is better than perfumed soap or shower gels.

PART TWO – COOKBOOK

Principles of the Cookbook

In this section we present more than two hundred recipes that are not only delicious but also good for health. We also include a new shopping list to help you restock your cupboard with lots of the foods that have been used in traditional medicine.

We have developed an exciting range of recipes based on the principles described in the previous section of the book. These are inspired by Asian and Mediterranean cooking to create a distinctive 'East meets West' style. The ready availability of ingredients for Asian and Mediterranean food now makes it easy for everyone to adopt this delicious, healthy way of eating. Asian-style recipes often look complicated because they have a lot of ingredients, many of which are spices and herbs, but don't let this put you off. If you have a tray of all your spices to hand it is only about adding a few ingredients – it doesn't add a lot of time or make the dish complicated – and remember spices are good for you.

The style of cooking used here ensures that fresh, wholesome ingredients are cooked in the healthiest way possible and served while everything is still fresh. Also we recommend that you:

- **Never use a microwave cooker, because free radicals are formed in the food**
- **Never use a pressure cooker, because it destroys vitamins and other important nutrients**

People today are very busy and they do not want to be relegated to the kitchen to cook for hours. However, this need not mean having to rely on junk processed food full of denatured ingredients and additives. Our aim is to make cooking simple and enjoyable and to provide healthy food.

CUSTOMISING THE RECIPES

All the recipes contain a full list of ingredients; use them as a guide and add or subtract ingredients to develop the meals that you like the most and, if appropriate, that are best suited to treating your illness.

Remember:

- Any vegetable can be replaced with others. Use your favourite, what's in season or what is in the fridge. For example, change asparagus for beans and vice versa.
- Although the recipes are based on measured quantities, there are no hard and fast rules. Use what is left in a packet, or omit ingredients if you do not like their taste. You can do this without significantly changing the recipe.
- Herbs and spices are a matter of taste, so vary the quantities to suit you. If you like spicy food we think you will enjoy the recipes as presented, but if you like milder food, simply cut down on the amount of spices, particularly chilli.
- Soya milk or cream can be substituted for dairy milk or cream in most other recipes, though all the recipes in this book already state this.
- Solid vegetable oil or grape-seed oil can substitute for butter to make pastry or cakes. Again, this substitution has already been made throughout these recipes.

Use your local farm shop or organic food supplier to help local industry, reduce transport miles, help the environment and help you.

The recipes previously published in *The Plant Programme* can be used to complement those in this book.

WEIGHTS AND MEASURES

All the recipes in this book are for four, unless otherwise stated. Conversions used are:

¼ cup = 60ml
½ cup = 125ml
1 cup = 250ml

1 tsp = 5ml
1 tbsp = 15ml

1oz = 30g
4oz = 125g
8oz = 250g
1lb = 500g

ESSENTIAL EQUIPMENT

We are assuming you have the usual range of cooking utensils, pots and pans, knives and so on. However, here are some things you may not have, that will help make the recipes easier to prepare:

- a **food processor** – there are many to choose from, the two most important functions to consider are chopping and puréeing
- a **garlic press**
- a **hand-held blender and food-processor attachment** – we find this the most useful piece of equipment in the kitchen; it is great for chopping small quantities of herbs, nuts, garlic or ginger, and for blending soups, making pastes, etc.
- an **ice-cream maker** (optional) – most of the sorbets and ice creams in this book have been made with a hand-turned ice-cream maker with a metal freezer bowl, which is kept in the freezer
- a **juice extractor**
- **metric measuring cups and spoons**
- a **microplane grater** – brilliant for grating ginger and lemon peel
- a **mincer** (optional) – if you want to mince your own ingredients this is a very useful piece of equipment (ours have a citrus squeezer and different-sized graters as attachments and we use them regularly)
- **pepper and salt mills**
- **sieves** – to rinse rice, drain pasta, strain soups, wash fruit, etc.
- a **salad shaker** – to dry salad vegetables easily, and prevent watering down the dressing
- a **char-grill pan** – a ridged, flat frying pan that is a quick and easy alternative to a barbecue, and is perfect for grilling prawns or squid and vegetables; large electric ones are now available
- a **sauté pan with lid**
- a **steamer with lid**
- a **non-stick wok with lid**

THE RESTOCKED CUPBOARD

This section gives an indicative shopping list, which includes most of the ingredients used in the recipes. You do not need to have everything, but it is particularly helpful to have the spices and herbs to hand.

When shopping, ensure that you read all labels carefully and avoid anything that contains milk solids, lactose, whey, casein, milk, yoghurt, cheese or other dairy ingredients. One brand of food may be dairy free, while another brand of the same food will contain dairy. For example, we have found that the traditional Indian bread, 'Naan', contains yoghurt if bought in large supermarkets, but not if you buy it from an Indian supermarket. We have found Japanese powdered dashi (soup stock) to contain lactose, even in Asian shops in Britain. The dairy additives are cheap fillers and would not be found in traditional Asian food.

THE ALKALINE-ACID HIERARCHY

We present our shopping list in order of increasing acid-generating potential: foods at the top of the list are highly alkaline and you can have plenty of them, while those at the bottom are the most acid and you should have them in moderation. All of these foods are now readily available at most supermarkets or, if you can't find them, try your nearest Asian grocery store.

1. Herbs and spices
2. Fruit and vegetables
3. Sugars
4. Beverages
5. Oils and fats
6. Legumes, nuts, seeds and grains
7. Fish, shellfish, meat, poultry and eggs

Herbs and spices

Fresh:

- Basil
- Bay leaves
- Chillies, red and green
- Chives

- Coriander (cilantro)
- Curry leaves (optional)
- Lemon grass (substitute with a whole lemon cut into quarters)
- Lime leaves
- Mint
- Parsley
- Rosemary
- Sage
- Thai basil (available from some Asian supermarkets)
- Thyme

Fresh herbs and spices, including garlic, ginger, chilli, lime leaves, lemon grass, parsley and bay leaves, can be frozen. Wrap them in foil and keep in the freezer until needed. They are best chopped or sliced while still frozen.

Dry:

- Bay leaves
- Black pepper
- Cardamom
- Cayenne or chilli powder
- Cinnamon, sticks and ground
- Cloves
- Ground coriander
- Ground cumin
- Garam masala
- Mustard seeds
- Nutmeg
- Paprika
- Saffron
- Sea salt
- Tamarind
- Turmeric

Bottled or canned:

- Curry paste
- Chilli sambal (minced chilli or sambal oelek)
- Thai sweet chilli sauce

Fruit

Any fresh fruit, including:

- Apples
- Bananas
- Berries
- Figs
- Grapefruit
- Grapes
- Kiwi fruit (Chinese gooseberry)
- Mandarins (clementines, tangerines)
- Mango
- Melon (cantaloupe, Galia)
- Nectarines
- Oranges
- Papaya
- Passion fruit
- Peaches
- Pears
- Pineapple
- Plums
- Pomegranate
- Pomelo
- Watermelon

Any frozen fruit, as long as it is without added sugar

Any freshly squeezed fruit juices

Dried fruit – buy the unsulphured varieties:

- Apricots
- Currants
- Dates
- Figs
- Prunes
- Raisins

Vegetables

Any fresh vegetable, including:

- Aubergine (eggplant)
- Avocado
- Bean sprouts
- Beetroot
- Bok choy
- Broccoli
- Cabbage
- Carrots
- Cauliflower
- Celeriac
- Celery
- Chicory (endive)
- *Choi sum*
- Corn on the cob, baby corn (sweet corn or maize)
- Cucumber
- Fennel
- Garlic
- Green beans
- Leeks
- Lettuce, all types
- Mangetout (snow peas)
- Mushrooms
- Mustard greens
- Onions, red and brown
- Parsnips
- Peppers, red, green, orange and yellow
- Potatoes
- Pumpkin
- Rocket
- Snap peas
- Spinach
- Sweet potato (kumara)
- Tomatoes, vine-ripened varieties
- Watercress
- Zucchini (courgette)

Frozen:

- Broad beans
- Corn
- Peas

Tinned or bottled:

- Artichokes in olive oil
- Bamboo shoots
- Water chestnuts

Dried:

- Chinese mushrooms
- Seaweed (kombu, wakame, nori)
- Shiitake mushrooms
- Sun-dried or sun-blush tomatoes

Sugars

- Dark chocolate (dairy free)
- Organic jams and marmalades (best made with fruit concentrate rather than sugar)
- Organic unrefined sugar or molasses
- Raw organic honey and maple syrup

Beverages

- Cider
- Filtered water and good-quality mineral waters in glass bottles
- Green tea
- Herb teas
- Pure cocoa
- Real ale and lagers
- Red and white wine

Oils and fats

- Grape-seed oil
- Olive oil
- Sesame oil
- Soya spread
- Sunflower spread
- Walnut oil

Legumes

- Bean curd (tofu, tempeh)
- Beans (cannellini, kidney, lima, soya etc.)
- Chickpeas
- Lentils
- Miso
- Split peas

Nuts

- Almonds
- Coconut
- Hazelnuts
- Pine nuts
- Walnuts

Seeds

- Pumpkin seeds
- Sesame seeds
- Sunflower seeds

Grains

- Barley
- Couscous
- Crispbreads
- Egg pasta and noodles
- Naan
- Oats
- Pastry
- Pitta bread
- Polenta
- Rice (arborio, basmati, sushi, wild)
- Rice noodles
- Spring roll wrappers
- Tortillas
- Wholemeal and rye breads
- Wholemeal and strong white/brown flour

Fish and seafood

All fish and seafood, including:

- Cod
- Crab
- Haddock
- Ocean trout
- Prawns
- Salmon (wild, not farmed)
- Scallops
- Sea bass
- Sole
- Squid
- Tuna

Meat, poultry and eggs (organic)

- Chicken
- Duck
- Eggs
- Lamb
- Pork
- Rabbit
- Venison

Sauces and seasonings

- Balsamic vinegar
- Capers
- Chinese cooking wine (substitute with dry sherry)
- Cider vinegar
- Fish sauce
- Furiyake Japanese seasoning
- Instant miso soup powder
- Light soya sauce (also shoyu and tamari sauce, some brands of which are gluten free)
- Mirin (substitute with Chinese cooking wine or medium sherry)
- Organic stock cubes (vegetable and chicken)
- Organic tomato ketchup
- Organic tomato paste
- Rice vinegar
- Teriyaki sauce
- Wasabi paste or powder
- Wine vinegar (red and white)

Good Beginnings

GUIDELINES

- *Freshly squeezed fruit and vegetable juices*
- *Fresh fruit salads*
- *Grilled vegetables and soups*
- *Muesli, oats, nuts and seeds*
- *Occasional eggs or fish*
- *Honey, molasses or raw cane sugar instead of refined white sugar*
- *Soya, coconut or rice milk to replace dairy milk*
- *Soya yoghurt and cream to replace dairy yoghurt or cream*

Breakfast is a matter of personal preference; some prefer only a light meal while for others breakfast is the most important meal of the day, but we recommend that everyone starts the day with a freshly squeezed fruit and/or vegetable juice, and follow that with a meal of their choice. If you like an egg or a piece of fish, serve it with potatoes or grilled vegetables rather than with bread. Here are a variety of ideas for a healthy start to the day.

FRUIT AND VEGETABLE JUICES

BANANA AND ORANGE MILK SHAKE
Serves 1–2
Preparation time: 1 minute

1 banana, peeled and sliced
⅓ cup fresh orange juice

1 cup soya milk
freshly grated nutmeg (optional)

1. Blend the banana, orange juice and soya milk with a hand-held blender or use a food processor
2. Serve sprinkled with grated nutmeg

KIWI, APPLE AND GINGER JUICE
Preparation time: 2–3 minutes

2 kiwi fruit, peeled and quartered
1 green apple, quartered
2cm piece fresh ginger, peeled

1. Put the fruit and ginger through a juicer and serve immediately (makes one cup)

MELON AND BANANA MILK SHAKE
Serves 1–2
Preparation time: 1–2 minutes

1 cup cantaloupe melon
1 small banana
⅓ cup orange juice
1 cup soya milk

1. Blend the fruit and soya milk with a hand-held blender or use a food processor; add a little more soya milk if it is too thick

RASPBERRY SMOOTHIE
Serves 1–2
Preparation time: 1–2 minutes

1 cup fresh orange or apple juice
½ cup fresh or frozen raspberries
1 small banana
1 tsp honey (optional)

1. Blend all the ingredients together using a hand-held blender or in a food processor

Variation: Replace raspberries with any other fruit

STRAWBERRY AND PEACH SHAKE
Serves 1–2
Preparation time: 1–2 minutes

1 cup strawberries
1 small peach, stoned and peeled
1 cup soya milk

1. Blend the fruit and soya milk with a hand-held blender or use a food processor; add a little more soya milk if it is too thick

TOMATO, RED PEPPER AND CUCUMBER JUICE
Serves 1
Preparation time: 2–3 minutes

4 tomatoes, halved
1 red pepper, seeded and sliced
¼ cucumber, cut into large pieces
1 large garlic clove, peeled
freshly ground black pepper
Tabasco sauce (optional)

1. Put the vegetables and garlic clove through a juicer, season to taste with black pepper and Tabasco sauce and serve immediately with some ice cubes

Fruit and vegetable juice suggestions:

Apple and celery juice
Cucumber, green pepper and pear juice
Grapefruit and celery juice
Kiwi, apple and mint juice
Orange, apple and raspberry juice
Papaya, banana and apple juice
Pineapple and peach juice
Tomato, carrot and celery juice

FRUIT TREATS

APPLE FRITTERS
Preparation time: 5–6 minutes
Cooking time: 6–8 minutes

2 tbsp raw cane sugar
1 tsp ground cinnamon
1 egg
½ cup plain flour
¼ cup soya milk
3–4 green apples, sliced and cored
grape-seed oil for frying

1. Mix the sugar and cinnamon together
2. Whisk together the egg and flour and add the soya milk to make a smooth paste
3. Dip the apple slices in the batter one at a time and shallow fry in the grape-seed oil until they are golden brown on both sides
4. Remove from the oil, drain on kitchen paper and sprinkle both sides with the cinnamon and sugar

APPLE TOAST
Serves 1
Preparation time: 1–2 minutes
Cooking time: 2 minutes

1 Granny Smith apple
1 tsp lemon juice
1–2 slices wholemeal bread, toasted
½ tsp ground cinnamon
1 tsp raw cane sugar (optional)

1. Grate the apple and toss it in the lemon juice

2. Top the toast with the grated apple and sprinkle with cinnamon and sugar

APRICOT COMPOTE
Preparation time: 1 minute
Cooking time: 10–15 minutes

200g dried apricots
2 tbsp sugar
½ tsp ground cinnamon
⅓ cup water
soya yoghurt

1. Put the apricots in a pan, sprinkle with the sugar and cinnamon, add the water and bring to a boil, then reduce the heat and simmer gently for 10–15 minutes
2. Serve with soya yoghurt or with porridge or muesli

BANANA TOAST
Serves 1
Preparation time: 1–2 minutes
Cooking time: 5–6 minutes

1–2 slices wholemeal bread
1 banana, peeled and mashed
½ tsp ground cinnamon
1 tsp brown sugar or honey

1. Toast the bread, top with the mashed banana and sprinkle with the cinnamon and brown sugar or honey
2. Grill for 3–4 minutes until the banana is warm and the sugar is caramelised

POACHED PEACHES WITH PORRIDGE
Preparation time: 5 minutes
Cooking time: 15–20 minutes

porridge oats
4–5 small peaches, stoned and cut into quarters
¼ cup raw cane sugar
1 tbsp lemon juice
soya milk or yoghurt

1. Cook the porridge oats following the instructions on the packet
2. Put the peaches in a saucepan with the sugar and lemon juice and 2 tablespoons water and simmer gently for about 10 minutes or until the peaches are soft
3. Serve the porridge with the peaches and some soya milk or yoghurt

Variation: use any soft fruit such as plums

STRAWBERRY, MELON AND KIWI FRUIT SALAD
Preparation time: 5–6 minutes

300g strawberries, sliced
½ Galia melon, cut into cubes
4 kiwis, peeled and sliced
1 tbsp lemon juice
soya yoghurt

1. Mix together the strawberries, melon and kiwi and sprinkle with lemon juice
2. Serve with soya yoghurt

STRAWBERRY AND RHUBARB COMPOTE
Preparation time: 5 minutes
Cooking time: 15 minutes

200g rhubarb, trimmed and cut into 2–3cm pieces
¼ cup raw cane sugar
¼ tsp ground cinnamon
1 vanilla bean or ¼ tsp vanilla essence
2 tbsp water
450g strawberries, halved
porridge or soya yoghurt

1. Put the rhubarb, sugar, cinnamon, vanilla bean and water in a saucepan, cover and simmer for about 15 minutes until the rhubarb is cooked, then remove from the heat and stir the strawberries through the mixture
2. Serve with porridge or soya yoghurt

SOMETHING SUBSTANTIAL

BANANA AND COCONUT PANCAKES

Preparation time: 10 minutes
Cooking time: 10 minutes

1 large egg
¼ cup sugar
½ cup self-raising flour
½ cup coconut milk
3–4 bananas, mashed
⅓ cup grape-seed oil
lemon juice

1. Lightly whisk together the egg and sugar, then fold in the sieved flour and coconut milk
2. Add the mashed banana and mix well
3. Heat the oil, add spoonfuls of the banana batter and fry both sides until the batter is cooked through and golden brown on both sides
4. Serve sprinkled with a little lemon juice

FRUIT MUFFINS

Preparation time: 5 minutes
Cooking time: 20–25 minutes

2 cups wholemeal flour
½ cup sugar
1 tbsp baking powder
¾–1 cup soya milk or fresh fruit juice
1 large egg
⅓ cup grape-seed oil
1 cup blueberries or chopped apple

1. Preheat the oven to 200°C
2. Lightly grease a muffin tin or line it with muffin cups

3. Sieve together the flour, sugar and baking powder
4. Lightly whisk together the soya milk, egg and oil, then gently fold in the flour ingredients (you don't need to mix them too well)
5. Add the blueberries or apple and again fold gently into the mixture
6. Divide the mixture between the muffin cups, filling them about two-thirds full
7. Bake for 20–25 minutes or until a toothpick inserted into the middle comes out clean
8. Allow to cool for 1 minute before removing from the pan

HOME-MADE SWISS MUESLI
Preparation time: 10 minutes
Cooking time: 1–2 minutes

¼ cup slivered almonds
¼ cup sesame seeds
¼ cup sunflower seeds
2 small Granny Smith apples
1 tsp lemon juice
1 ½ cups fresh apple or orange juice
1 cup raisins
1 cup soya yoghurt
2 tsp honey (optional) or to taste
2 cups rolled oats
1 tsp ground cinnamon
¼ tsp ground nutmeg
1 punnet blueberries

1. Toast the almonds, sesame and sunflower seeds in the oven or in a pan for a few minutes
2. Grate the apple and toss in the lemon juice
3. Mix all the ingredients, except the blueberries, together, cover and refrigerate overnight (this is actually quite delicious after soaking for only about 10 minutes)
4. Serve with extra soya yoghurt or milk and fresh blueberries

HOME-MADE TOASTED MUESLI
Preparation time: 10 minutes
Cooking time: 45 minutes

½ cup apple juice
1 cup dried apricots, cut into slivers
200g raisins
½ cup desiccated coconut
300g rolled oats
½ cup almonds or hazelnuts
½ cup sunflower seeds
½ cup pumpkin seeds
¼ cup sesame seeds
2 tbsp grape-seed oil

1. Preheat the oven to 180°C
2. Mix together all the ingredients in a large oven-proof dish
3. Bake in the oven until the oats are a light brown colour (about 45 minutes), stirring the mixture every 15 minutes to avoid the bottom layer burning
4. Turn off the oven and leave the muesli in the oven until it cools

Serve with some fresh fruit and soya milk or yoghurt

Store in a dry cool place in an airtight container for up to a month

SOMETHING SAVOURY

AVOCADO AND TOMATO SALSA ON TOAST
Preparation time: 10 minutes
Cooking time: 2–3 minutes

4 slices Italian bread
1–2 garlic cloves, peeled

1 small avocado, halved and stone removed
1 tsp lemon juice
4 medium vine-ripened tomatoes, chopped
½ cup fresh coriander, chopped
freshly ground black pepper

1. Toast the bread then rub a garlic clove over one side
2. Scoop the flesh out of the avocado and toss with a little lemon juice, then gently stir through the tomatoes and coriander and season with black pepper
3. Serve on top of the toast

CORN AND PEPPER FRITTERS
Preparation time: 5 minutes
Cooking time: 15–20 minutes

1 large egg
½ cup plain flour
¼ cup water or soya milk
2 garlic cloves, crushed
1 tsp chilli sambal or ½ red chilli, sliced (optional)
1 cup fresh coriander, chopped
1 small green or red pepper, seeded and diced
1 small red onion, diced
1 cup sweet corn kernels
vegetable oil for shallow frying

1. Whisk the egg, add the flour and a little water or soya milk to make a thick batter, then stir through the garlic and chilli
2. In a separate bowl mix together the coriander, pepper, red onion and sweet corn, then add them to the batter and stir to mix thoroughly
3. Heat the oil and add small spoonfuls of the vegetables; flatten the balls slightly and cook, turning occasionally until golden brown each side and cooked through but still soft in the middle

These are delicious served with Thai sweet chilli dipping sauce.

FRIED RICE

If you have leftover rice this is a very easy and tasty start to the day. We often have it for Sunday breakfast.

Preparation time: 5–10 minutes
Cooking time: 10–15 minutes

2 tbsp olive oil
3–4 garlic cloves, sliced
1 tbsp fresh ginger, grated
1 red chilli, sliced
1 red pepper, diced
1 cup fresh or frozen peas
1 cup fresh or frozen sweet-corn kernels
8 baby mushrooms, sliced
4 spring onions, thinly sliced
1–2 tbsp soya sauce
1 tbsp Chinese cooking wine
1–2 cups cooked rice
½ cup fresh coriander, chopped
freshly ground black pepper
4 eggs (optional)

1. Heat a wok or saucepan, add the oil and stir-fry the garlic, ginger and chilli for about 30 seconds
2. Add the red pepper (and peas and sweet corn, if fresh) and continue to stir-fry for about a minute, then add the mushrooms, spring onions, 1 tablespoon soya sauce and the cooking wine and cook for another 1–2 minutes
3. Add the cooked rice (and peas and sweet corn, if frozen), stir to mix thoroughly and continue to cook until the rice and vegetables are heated through, then stir through the fresh coriander; add a little extra soya sauce to taste and season with black pepper
4. While the rice is heating through, poach the eggs until they are cooked to your liking

Divide the rice between four bowls and serve with an egg on top and a little chilli sauce on the side.

GRILLED BALSAMIC MUSHROOMS ON TOAST
Preparation time: 5 minutes
Cooking time: 5 minutes

8 large mushrooms
1–2 tbsp balsamic vinegar
4 slices bread, toasted
2 tbsp fresh flat-leaf parsley, chopped
freshly ground black pepper

1. Peel the mushrooms and remove the stalk
2. Sprinkle a little balsamic vinegar over each mushroom and grill until cooked through
3. Serve on toast; sprinkle with chopped parsley and season with black pepper

Variation: spread toast with pesto (page 233) or olive tapenade (page 233)

MUSHROOM, SPINACH AND TOMATO BRUSCHETTA
Preparation time: 5 minutes
Cooking time: 6–8 minutes

4 slices Italian bread
4 tbsp olive oil
2 garlic cloves, peeled
1 tsp chilli sambal (optional)
1 tsp freshly ground black pepper
4 large flat mushrooms, peeled
50g baby spinach leaves
1 large vine-ripened tomato, finely diced
2 tbsp chopped coriander
freshly ground black pepper

1. Lightly brush both sides of the bread with half the oil and grill both sides until golden brown, then rub a garlic clove over one side
2. Add the chilli and black pepper to the remaining oil, spoon it over the mushrooms and grill for 3–4 minutes or until the mushrooms are cooked
3. Top the toasted bread with fresh spinach leaves, the grilled mushroom and diced tomato, sprinkle with chopped coriander and season with black pepper

SCRAMBLED EGGS WITH GARLIC AND SPRING ONIONS
Preparation time: 5 minutes
Cooking time: 4–5 minutes

6 eggs
2 tbsp soya cream
freshly ground black pepper
2 tsp olive oil
8 spring onions, finely sliced
3–4 garlic cloves, minced
1 green chilli (optional)
fresh parsley, chopped

1. Lightly beat together the eggs and soya cream and season with black pepper
2. Heat the oil and stir-fry the spring onions, garlic and chilli for 1–2 minutes
3. Add the egg mixture and stir over a medium heat until the egg is cooked to your liking and serve garnished with the chopped parsley

Variation: replace the spring onions with finely chopped leek

SWEET POTATO FRITTERS WITH POACHED EGGS
Preparation time: 10 minutes
Cooking time: 10–15 minutes

200g sweet potato, peeled and grated
½ cup plain flour
1 large egg
2–3 tbsp soya milk
freshly ground black pepper
¼ cup vegetable oil
4 medium eggs

1. Whisk together the flour, the large egg and enough soya milk to make a thick batter; add the sweet potato and season with black pepper, stir to mix thoroughly; divide the potato mixture into smallish balls and flatten slightly
2. Heat the oil and add the sweet potato balls in batches to the pan and shallow fry until they are nicely browned, then turn the potato

over and cook the other side (add a little more oil if necessary); drain the fritters on kitchen paper and keep warm if necessary

3. Meanwhile, half-fill a frying pan with water and when gently simmering, break the eggs into individual poaching rings and cook for about 3 minutes or until done to your liking
4. Drain the eggs and serve on top of the potatoes

ZUCCHINI FRITTERS
Preparation time: 5–10 minutes
Cooking time: 6–8 minutes

1 large egg
½ cup plain flour
½–1 cup soya milk
2 medium zucchini, grated
freshly ground black pepper
¼ cup vegetable oil

1. Whisk together the egg and flour and gradually add enough soya milk to make a thick smooth batter
2. Stir through the zucchini and season with black pepper
3. Heat the oil and add spoonfuls of the zucchini batter, flatten slightly and cook until they are golden brown on both sides but still soft in the middle

These are delicious served with sweet chilli dipping sauce

BREAKFAST SOUPS

BEAN CURD AND SPINACH MISO SOUP
Preparation time: 5 minutes
Cooking time: 5 minutes

120g soft bean curd, drained
1 litre chicken stock
4 spring onions, sliced diagonally
100g baby spinach leaves
½ cup bean sprouts
1 tbsp light soya sauce

4 tbsp miso paste
fresh coriander leaves, coarsely chopped
freshly ground black pepper

1. Cut the bean curd into thin slices
2. Bring the stock to a gentle simmer, then add the spring onions, spinach, bean sprouts and soya sauce and simmer gently for 1–2 minutes until the spinach has just wilted
3. Take the soup off the heat, add the miso and stir to dissolve (this can be done using a small sieve or tea strainer which removes the coarse fibres)
4. Divide the bean curd and a few coriander leaves among four serving bowls, then pour over the soup and season with black pepper

CHICKEN AND SNOW PEA NOODLE SOUP
Preparation time: 5 minutes
Cooking time: 10–15 minutes

150g thin egg noodles
1 litre chicken stock
1 star anise
2cm piece fresh ginger, thinly sliced
2 chicken breasts, thinly sliced
6–8 oyster mushrooms, sliced
1 tbsp Chinese cooking wine
2 tbsp soya sauce
4–6 spring onions, sliced
60g mangetout
1 tbsp sesame oil
1 cup baby spinach leaves
fresh coriander leaves

1. Bring a pan of water to the boil, add the noodles and cook according to the instructions on the packet, then drain and keep warm if necessary
2. Heat the stock with the star anise, ginger and chicken and simmer gently for 5–6 minutes
3. Add the mushrooms, Chinese cooking wine and soya sauce and continue to simmer for 2–3 minutes, then add the spring

onions, mangetout and sesame oil and simmer for another 1–2 minutes

4. Divide the cooked noodles, spinach leaves and fresh coriander among the soup plates and spoon over the chicken soup

Meals on the Run

GUIDELINES

- *Delicious soups based on fresh vegetables*
- *Lots of different raw fresh salad vegetables and fruit*
- *Cheese replaced with home-made dips and spreads*
- *Dairy-free bread, oat and rice cakes*
- *Freshly shelled nuts, seeds and dried fruits*

Many people's busy lifestyles mean that they and their families frequently eat ready-made meals and snacks, especially at lunch-time. Relying on plastic wrapped sandwiches, indifferent salads or reheated chips is not good for anyone's health. In this section we have put together some ideas for delicious light meals that will stop you reaching for those old staples cheese and yoghurt. All of the recipes in this section are, of course, equally as good as a starter or as a main evening meal.

SUPER SOUPS

Soups are a great way of ensuring you eat lots of vegetables. Many of these soups are nutritious meals in themselves or they make delicious starters for main meals and dinner parties. They can be heated up and many of them are as tasty cold as hot, so can be taken to the office for lunch.

AVOCADO SOUP
Preparation time: 10 minutes
Cooking time: 15 minutes

40g slivered almonds (optional)
2 large ripe avocados
¼ cup lemon juice
1 litre chicken stock
3–4 garlic cloves, sliced
1 green chilli, sliced
1–2 tbsp chopped fresh mint
freshly ground black pepper
2 tbsp fresh coriander

1. Toast the almonds under a grill or in the oven for a few minutes until they turn golden (watch them carefully so they do not burn)
2. Peel and stone the avocados and purée with a little of the lemon juice
3. Heat the stock with the garlic and chilli and simmer for 10 minutes
4. Add the avocado to the stock and whisk to mix in, bring the soup back to a very gentle simmer (do not boil), then add the remaining lemon juice and mint; season with black pepper and serve garnished with fresh coriander and the toasted almonds

BROAD BEAN AND LETTUCE SOUP
Preparation time: 10 minutes
Cooking time: 30–35 minutes

2 tbsp olive oil
1 medium onion, peeled and coarsely chopped
4–5 garlic cloves, chopped

1 green chilli (optional)
1 medium potato, peeled and coarsely chopped
2 cups fresh or frozen broad beans
1 large romaine lettuce, washed and coarsely shredded
1 ¼ litres chicken or vegetable stock
½ cup fresh flat-leaf parsley
¼ cup fresh mint leaves
freshly ground black pepper

1. Heat the olive oil, add the onion and gently sauté for about 2–3 minutes until the onion is translucent
2. Add the garlic and chilli and sauté for another minute, then add the potato, broad beans and lettuce and stir to coat in the oil
3. Add the stock, cover and simmer gently for about 20 minutes or until the potato is soft
4. Purée the soup, return to the heat if necessary and bring back to a simmer
5. Stir through the mint and parsley and season with black pepper

BROCCOLI AND POTATO SOUP
Preparation time: 10 minutes
Cooking time: 30–35 minutes

4 tbsp olive oil
1 large onion, peeled and chopped
3–4 garlic cloves, chopped
500g potatoes, cleaned and diced
400g broccoli, cut into small florets, the stalks peeled and chopped
1 ¼ litres stock
freshly ground black pepper
fresh basil leaves, coarsely chopped

1. Sauté the onion in the olive oil for 3–4 minutes, add the garlic and continue to sauté for another minute
2. Add the potatoes and broccoli, stir and sauté for another 1–2 minutes
3. Add the stock, season to taste with black pepper, bring to a slow simmer, cover and continue to simmer for 20–25 minutes

until the potatoes are soft and beginning to break up, then stir through the basil leaves

Variation: use 1 tbsp pesto (page 233) instead of the basil leaves

CAULIFLOWER SOUP
Preparation time: 10 minutes
Cooking time: 20–25 minutes

1 onion, coarsely chopped
1 cauliflower, cut into smallish florets
2 celery stalks, chopped
3–4 garlic cloves, chopped
1 ½ litres chicken or vegetable stock
2 tbsp soya sauce
1–2 tbsp brown rice vinegar* to taste (optional)
fresh flat-leaf parsley

1. Put all the vegetables and the garlic into a large saucepan, add the stock and simmer for about 20–25 minutes until the cauliflower is soft and you can mash it with a fork
2. Add the soya sauce and briefly purée the soup until it is coarsely blended
3. Serve into soup bowls then stir through some brown rice vinegar and chopped parsley

*If you like Worcester sauce you could use this instead, but use sparingly as it is very strong

CRAB AND SWEET CORN SOUP
Preparation time: 10 minutes
Cooking time: 15 minutes

2 tbsp olive oil
1 tbsp fresh ginger, grated
4 spring onions, finely sliced
1 litre chicken stock
2 cups fresh or frozen sweet corn kernels, coarsely chopped in the food processor
1 tbsp mirin or Chinese cooking wine
2 tbsp light soya sauce

1 can white crab meat, rinsed, drained and flaked
1 tsp cornflour
1 egg
2 tsp sesame oil
2 tsp brown rice vinegar
½ cup fresh coriander, chopped

1. Heat the olive oil and stir-fry the ginger and spring onions for about a minute
2. Add the chicken stock, sweet corn, mirin and soya sauce and simmer for 2–3 minutes, then add the crab and continue to simmer for another 2 minutes
3. Mix the cornflour with a little water to make a thin paste and pour this into the soup and simmer for 2 minutes
4. Lightly beat the egg with the sesame oil
5. Remove the soup from the heat, add the vinegar, and pour in the beaten egg slowly, stirring gently
6. Serve immediately, garnished with coriander

Variation: use 2 poached chicken breasts, shredded, instead of the crab, and add with the stock

CURRIED CHICKEN NOODLE SOUP
Preparation time: 10 minutes (40 minutes including marinating time)
Cooking time: 10–15 minutes

2–3 chicken breasts, skinned and sliced
3–4 tbsp olive oil
2 tbsp light soya sauce
8 dried Chinese or shiitake mushrooms
150g dried thin egg noodles
4 garlic cloves, crushed
1 tbsp grated fresh ginger
1 red chilli, sliced
2 tbsp curry powder
1½ litres chicken stock
350g broccoli, cut into small florets
4–6 spring onions, sliced
fresh coriander, chopped

1. Marinate the chicken with 2 tablespoons olive oil and the soya sauce for at least 30 minutes
2. Pour boiling water over the mushrooms and leave them to soak for 30 minutes
3. Cook the noodles in plenty of boiling water according to the instructions on the packet, then drain and keep warm
4. Pan-fry the chicken in the marinade until it is just cooked, remove from the pan and keep warm
5. Heat the remaining olive oil and sauté the garlic, ginger, chilli and curry powder for 1 minute
6. Add the stock and the mushrooms together with the liquid they have been soaked in and simmer for about 3–4 minutes
7. Add the broccoli and continue to simmer for another 3–4 minutes, then add the spring onions and cook for another minute
8. Divide the noodles among four serving bowls, top with the sliced chicken, ladle over the soup and vegetables and garnish with fresh coriander

FENNEL SOUP WITH PRAWNS
Preparation time: 10 minutes
Cooking time: 25–30 minutes

3 tbsp olive oil
2 leeks, washed and finely sliced
4–5 garlic cloves, chopped
2 large fennel bulbs, chopped, leaves retained if available
1 ½ litres chicken or vegetable stock
200g raw tiger prawns, peeled and rinsed
fresh tarragon
freshly ground black pepper

1. Heat the olive oil and sauté the leeks for about 3–4 minutes until soft and translucent
2. Add the garlic and fennel, stir to coat in the oil and continue to sauté for another 1–2 minutes, then add the stock and simmer for 15–20 minutes until the fennel is soft; allow the soup to cool slightly, then purée in a food processor before pouring the soup through a sieve to remove the coarse fennel fibres

3. Return the soup to the pan, bring to a gentle simmer, add the prawns and cook for a further 3–4 minutes until the prawns have just turned pink
4. Serve garnished with fresh tarragon or chopped fennel leaves and season with black pepper

GINGERED BROCCOLI AND LEMON GRASS SOUP
Preparation time: 10 minutes
Cooking time: 20 minutes

3 tbsp olive oil
1 large brown onion, coarsely chopped
3–4 garlic cloves, chopped
1 heaped tbsp grated fresh ginger
1 green chilli, sliced
1 stalk lemon grass, cut into 2½cm lengths
2–3 lime leaves
500g broccoli, coarsely chopped and stems peeled
1½ litres vegetable or chicken stock
2 tbsp lemon juice
freshly ground black pepper

1. Heat the olive oil and sauté the onion for 3–4 minutes
2. Add the garlic, ginger, chilli, lemon grass and lime leaves and continue to sauté for another minute
3. Add the broccoli and stir to coat in the oil, then add the stock and simmer for about 10–15 minutes or until the broccoli is soft
4. Remove the lime leaves and lemon grass and purée the soup; return to heat if necessary and just before serving stir through the lemon juice and season with black pepper

GINGERED CARROT AND CUMIN SOUP
Preparation time: 10–15 minutes
Cooking time: 30 minutes

2 tbsp olive oil
2 medium leeks, washed and coarsely sliced
2–3 garlic cloves, chopped
1 heaped tbsp grated fresh ginger

1 tbsp ground cumin
500g carrots, sliced
1 ¼ litres chicken or vegetable stock
juice of 2 oranges
1–2 tbsp chopped fresh flat-leaf parsley

1. Heat the olive oil in a large saucepan, add the leeks and sauté for 2–3 minutes, then add the garlic, ginger and ground cumin and continue to sauté for another minute
2. Add the carrots and stir to coat in the oil and spices and sauté for another 2 minutes
3. Pour over the hot stock, add the orange juice, cover and simmer gently for about 20–25 minutes until the carrots are soft
4. Purée the soup until smooth, reheat if necessary and serve garnished with parsley and sprinkled with a little extra ground cumin if desired

INDONESIAN CHICKEN NOODLE SOUP (LAKSA)

Don't be put off by the long list of ingredients; they are mostly spices and a mixture of vegetables.

Preparation time: 15 minutes
Cooking time: 25 minutes

2 chicken breasts, skinned
3–4 garlic cloves, crushed
1 tbsp ginger
1 red or green chilli, sliced
1 tbsp ground cumin
1 tbsp ground coriander
1 ½ tsp turmeric
1 ½ tsp cayenne pepper
1 onion, peeled and coarsely chopped
6 blanched almonds
1 tsp shrimp paste
2 tbsp olive oil
1 stalk lemon grass, cut into 2cm slices
3–4 lime leaves
1 litre chicken or vegetable stock

400ml coconut milk
2–3 tbsp fresh lime juice
2 tbsp fish sauce
¼ tsp palm or brown sugar (optional)
6 spring onions, sliced
12 mangetout, cut in half
½ cup bamboo shoots
150g spinach or rocket
¼ cup fresh mint leaves, chopped
100g thin rice vermicelli noodles
1 cup bean sprouts
½ cup fresh coriander, chopped

1. Poach the chicken breasts until they are just cooked through, then drain and slice and keep warm
2. Put the garlic, ginger, chilli, cumin, coriander, turmeric, cayenne pepper, onion, almonds, shrimp paste and ½ cup of the stock in a blender and process to a smooth paste
3. Heat the olive oil, add the lemon grass, lime leaves and paste and fry for 3–4 minutes, stirring continuously to prevent it sticking, then add the remaining stock and simmer for about 15 minutes
4. Add the coconut milk, lime juice, fish sauce and sugar and simmer gently for another 5 minutes
5. Add the spring onions, mangetout, bamboo shoots, spinach and mint and simmer for another 1–2 minutes or until the spinach has just wilted
6. Meanwhile, put the rice noodles in a bowl, pour over boiling water and leave to stand for about 3–5 minutes, then drain
7. Divide the rice noodles among four large soup bowls, top with some fresh bean sprouts, the sliced chicken and fresh coriander and ladle over the soup

MISO SOUP WITH BEAN CURD AND SPINACH
Preparation time: 5 minutes
Cooking time: 15 minutes

120g bean curd, cut into cubes
½ cup baby spinach leaves
4 spring onions, sliced

1 litre chicken stock
2–3 garlic cloves, crushed
1 stalk lemon grass, cut into 3–4 slices and slightly crushed
4–5 lime leaves
1 tbsp grated fresh ginger
1 tsp black pepper
4 tbsp miso
fresh coriander

1. Divide the bean curd, spinach and spring onions among four soup bowls
2. Simmer the chicken stock with the garlic, lemon grass, lime leaves, ginger and black pepper for about 15 minutes
3. Take off the heat, remove the lime leaves and lemon grass and stir in the miso paste (this can be done by putting the miso in a tea strainer or small sieve, which sieves out the coarse fibres)
4. Pour the soup over the bean curd and spinach and garnish with fresh coriander

PEA AND BROAD BEAN SOUP
Preparation time: 15–20 minutes
Cooking time: 25–30 minutes

200g fresh or frozen peas
400g fresh or frozen broad beans
3 tbsp olive oil
2 medium red onions, chopped
4 garlic cloves, chopped
2 medium potatoes, peeled and finely chopped
3 cups chicken stock
½ cup fresh mint leaves, chopped
½ cup fresh basil, shredded
freshly ground black pepper

1. Thaw the frozen peas and beans if necessary and peel the broad beans (although this takes a little bit of time and is a bit fiddly, it is well worth the effort)
2. Heat the olive oil and sauté the onion for about 5 minutes until it is soft and translucent, add the garlic and sauté for another minute, then add the potatoes and fresh peas and beans and stir to coat in the oil

3. Add the stock and simmer gently for about 20 minutes until the potato is cooked through adding frozen peas and/or beans after about 10 minutes

4. Coarsely purée the soup (it should be quite thick), then stir through the mint and basil and season with black pepper; reheat if necessary

PRAWN AND MUSHROOM SOUP

Preparation time: 10 minutes
Cooking time: 10 minutes

12–16 medium raw tiger prawns, peeled and washed
1 tbsp sesame oil
2–3 garlic cloves, crushed
1 tbsp fresh ginger, grated
1 red chilli, finely chopped
150g fresh shiitake or chestnut mushrooms, sliced
1 litre chicken stock
1 tbsp mirin or Chinese cooking wine
1 tbsp Chinese rice vinegar
1 cup baby spinach leaves
4–5 spring onions, finely sliced
2 tbsp chopped fresh coriander
freshly ground black pepper

1. Bring a little bit of water to a rolling boil, add the prawns, turn off the heat and leave the prawns for 2–3 minutes to turn pink, then drain (if you are using precooked prawns omit this step)
2. In a separate saucepan, heat the sesame oil and sauté the garlic, ginger and chilli for one minute
3. Add the mushrooms and continue to sauté for another 2 minutes
4. Add the chicken stock, mirin (or Chinese cooking wine) and Chinese rice vinegar and bring to a gentle simmer
5. Add the prawns, spinach and spring onions and continue to simmer until the leaves are just wilted (1–2 minutes)
6. Divide the soup among the serving bowls, garnish with fresh coriander and season with black pepper

Variation: use bean curd instead of prawns; fry the bean curd separately in a little sesame oil, cut into cubes and divide among the soup plates, then pour over the soup

PRAWN LAKSA
Don't be put off by the long list of ingredients, they are mostly spices and vegetables.

Preparation time: 15 minutes
Cooking time: 20 minutes

4–5 garlic cloves
1 tbsp fresh ginger
1 tbsp ground cumin
1 tbsp ground coriander
½ tsp ground turmeric
1 red chilli, sliced
1 stalk lemon grass
1 tsp shrimp paste
2 tbsp olive oil
1 litre vegetable or chicken stock
1 fresh lemon, quartered
1 cup coconut milk
3–4 lime leaves
2 tbsp lime juice
2 tbsp fish sauce
350g raw prawns
16 baby sweet corn, halved
1 cup peas
2 small bok choy, quartered
4–5 spring onions, sliced
16 mangetout
1 cup bean sprouts
100g rocket
100g rice vermicelli noodles
½ cup fresh coriander, chopped
freshly ground black pepper

1. Process the garlic, ginger, cumin, coriander, turmeric, chilli, lemon grass and shrimp paste with a little of the stock to a smooth paste in a food processor or blender

197

2. Heat the olive oil in a saucepan or wok and fry the paste for 2–3 minutes, stirring to ensure it doesn't burn

3. Add the stock and lemon and simmer gently for about 10–15 minutes

4. Add the coconut milk, lime leaves, lime juice and fish sauce and simmer for about 5 minutes

5. Add the prawns, sweet corn, peas and bok choy to the stock and continue to simmer for another 3–4 minutes until the prawns turn pink

6. Add the spring onions, mangetout, bean sprouts and rocket and simmer for another minute or until the rocket has just wilted

7. Meanwhile put the rice noodles in a bowl, pour over boiling water and leave to stand for about 4–5 minutes, then drain and keep warm

8. Divide the rice noodles between four large soup bowls, and pour over the soup, dividing the prawns and vegetables among the dishes, garnish with fresh coriander and season with black pepper

PUMPKIN SOUP

Preparation time: 15 minutes
Cooking time: 35 minutes

2 tbsp olive oil
1 onion, chopped
1 leek, sliced
3–4 garlic cloves, chopped
2 tsp ground cumin
2 tsp ground coriander
1 large pumpkin, peeled, seeded and chopped
1¼ litres chicken or vegetable stock
1 tsp black pepper
fresh coriander or parsley
freshly grated nutmeg

1. Heat the olive oil in a large saucepan, add the onion and leek and sauté for 2–3 minutes, then add the garlic, ground cumin and coriander and continue to sauté for another minute

2. Add the pumpkin, stir to coat in the oil and continue to sauté for another minute, then pour over the stock, cover and simmer gently for about 30 minutes until the pumpkin is soft

3. Remove from the heat and purée until smooth; reheat if necessary, season with black pepper and garnish with fresh parsley or coriander and a grating of fresh nutmeg

Variation: use sweet potato

RED PEPPER AND LENTIL SOUP
Preparation time: 15 minutes
Cooking time: 35–40 minutes

2 tbsp olive oil
1 onion, peeled and coarsely chopped
3–4 garlic cloves, sliced
1 tbsp fresh ginger, grated
1 red chilli, sliced
1 stalk lemon grass, cut into 3–4 pieces and slightly crushed
3–4 lime leaves
½ cup red lentils
2 medium red peppers, seeded and coarsely chopped
1¼ litres chicken or vegetable stock
2 tbsp brown rice vinegar
2 tbsp light soya sauce
freshly ground black pepper
fresh coriander leaves

1. Heat the olive oil in a saucepan, add the onion and sauté for 2–3 minutes until the onion has become translucent

2. Add the garlic, ginger, chilli, lemon grass, lime leaves and red lentils, stir to coat in the oil and continue to sauté for another minute

3. Add the red peppers, stir to coat in the oil then add the hot stock, cover and leave to simmer gently for about 30 minutes or until the lentils are soft

4. Remove the lemon grass and lime leaves and blend the soup until smooth

5. Stir through the rice vinegar and soya sauce, reheat if necessary, then season with black pepper and garnish with fresh coriander

SPICY CHICKEN NOODLE SOUP

Preparation time: 10 minutes
Cooking time: 20 minutes

1 ½ litres chicken stock
4–5 garlic cloves, crushed
1 tbsp grated fresh ginger
2 long green chillies, finely sliced
2–3 lime leaves
1 stalk lemon grass, sliced into 3–4 pieces
1 tsp coarse black pepper
1 whole lemon, cut into quarters
2 chicken thighs
100g rice noodles
6 spring onions, sliced
200g bok choy, quartered
1 cup bean sprouts
½ cup fresh coriander leaves

1. Heat the stock in a large saucepan, add the garlic, ginger, chillies, lime leaves, lemon grass, black pepper and lemon, cover and leave to simmer gently for about 15 minutes
2. In a separate pan gently poach the chicken for about 10 minutes until it is just cooked through, then drain and cut into slices
3. Cut the noodles into 4cm lengths, put into a bowl, pour over boiling water and leave for approximately 5 minutes until they are soft (or according to the instructions on the packet), then drain and keep warm
4. Remove the lemon grass, lime leaves and lemon from the soup and return to the heat
5. Add the spring onions, bok choy and chicken and simmer for another 2–3 minutes until the vegetables are just soft
6. Divide the noodles and bean sprouts between the individual soup bowls, top with the bean sprouts, then pour over the soup and garnish with fresh coriander

SPICY LENTIL SOUP WITH BEAN SPROUTS
Preparation time: 10 minutes
Cooking time: 35–45 minutes

1 tbsp tamarind pulp
2 tbsp olive oil
1 large brown onion, coarsely chopped
4–5 garlic cloves, sliced
1 tbsp grated fresh ginger
1 tsp ground cumin
1 tsp ground coriander
½ tsp ground turmeric
1 tsp cayenne pepper
1 cup green lentils, washed
1 cup coconut milk
1 ½ litres chicken or vegetable stock
1 cup bean sprouts
½ cup cooked rice
fresh coriander

1. Soak the tamarind pulp in ¼ cup of boiling water for about 15 minutes, then drain, reserving the liquid; squeeze the pulp to extract all the tamarind
2. Heat the olive oil and fry the onion for 3–4 minutes, then add the garlic and ginger and all the dry spices, and continue to stir-fry for another 1–2 minutes
3. Add the lentils and stir to coat in the oil, then add the coconut milk and bring to a gentle simmer; pour in the stock and simmer gently for about 30 minutes until the lentils are soft
4. Purée the soup and return it to the pan, then add the cooked rice and reheat
5. Divide the bean sprouts among the soup plates, pour over the soup and serve garnished with fresh coriander

SPICY FISH SOUP
Preparation time: 15 minutes plus 15 minutes to marinate
Cooking time: 15–20 minutes

3 tbsp light soya sauce
1 tsp ground cumin

½ tsp cayenne pepper
200g swordfish or other firm white fish, cut into cubes
2 tbsp olive oil
1 small leek, finely sliced
1 small fennel bulb, finely sliced
1 tbsp crushed garlic
1 tbsp grated fresh ginger
1 red chilli, sliced
1 litre chicken or vegetable stock
1 tbsp mirin or Chinese cooking wine
8 oyster mushrooms, sliced
4–6 spring onions, sliced
1 tbsp chopped fresh tarragon
½ cup fresh flat-leaf parsley
freshly ground black pepper

1. Mix together the soya sauce, cumin and cayenne pepper, pour over the fish and leave to marinate for 15 minutes
2. Heat the olive oil and add the fish and the marinade and gently sauté the fish for 3–4 minutes until it is just cooked, then remove from the pan and keep warm
3. Add the leek and fennel to the pan and sauté for 3–4 minutes until they are soft (add a little more olive oil if necessary), then add the garlic, ginger and chilli and continue to sauté for another minute
4. Add the stock and mirin and bring to a gentle simmer, then add the oyster mushrooms and simmer for 5 minutes
5. Add the fish, spring onions and tarragon to the stock and continue to simmer for another 1–2 minutes
6. Serve garnished with fresh parsley and season with black pepper

SPICY TOMATO SOUP
Preparation time: 10 minutes
Cooking time: 25 minutes

2 tbsp olive oil
1 red onion, coarsely chopped
2–3 garlic cloves, chopped
1 stalk lemon grass, cut into 4 or 5 pieces

4 lime leaves
8–10 curry leaves (optional)
1 tsp ground cumin
½ red chilli or 1 tsp cayenne pepper
400g vine-ripened tomatoes, coarsely chopped
1½ litres chicken or vegetable stock
2 tbsp fresh lime or lemon juice
1 tsp coarse black pepper
freshly chopped coriander

1. Heat the olive oil in a large saucepan; add the onion and sauté for 2–3 minutes
2. Add the garlic, lemon grass, lime leaves, curry leaves, ground cumin and chilli and sauté for another minute, then add the tomatoes, stir briefly, then pour over the stock
3. Simmer gently for about 15–20 minutes until the tomatoes are soft
4. Remove the lemon grass and lime leaves and purée the soup until smooth
5. Reheat if necessary, stir in the lime or lemon juice and serve garnished with fresh coriander

SWEET POTATO AND YAM SOUP
This is helpful if you suffer from premenstrual or menopausal symptoms. Yams are readily available in Asian grocery shops and increasingly in some supermarkets.

Preparation time: 10–15 minutes
Cooking time: 25–30 minutes

2 tbsp olive oil
1 medium brown onion, roughly chopped
1 leek, washed and sliced
4–5 garlic cloves, chopped or sliced
3–4 lime leaves
1 red chilli, sliced
500g sweet potato, peeled and diced
500g yam, peeled and diced
1½ litres chicken stock
1 lemon, cut into 8 wedges

freshly ground black pepper
fresh coriander leaves

1. Heat the olive oil and sauté the onion and leek for 2–3 minutes, then add the garlic, lime leaves and chilli and continue to sauté for another minute
2. Add the sweet potato and yam, stir to coat in the oil and sauté for a minute, then pour over the stock, add the lemon and simmer for about 20–25 minutes until the vegetables are soft
3. Remove the lime leaves and lemon and purée the soup until smooth
4. Season with black pepper and garnish with fresh coriander

THAI-STYLE COCONUT AND PRAWN SOUP
Preparation time: 5 minutes
Cooking time: 12–15 minutes

1 litre chicken stock
6–8 lime leaves
2 stalks lemon grass, cut into 3–4 pieces and crushed slightly
1 red chilli
2cm piece of fresh ginger, peeled and thinly sliced
1 cup coconut milk
3 tsp fish sauce
2–3 field mushrooms, sliced
10–12 green beans, topped, tailed and halved
300g green tiger prawns, peeled
8–12 mangetout, halved
4 spring onions, sliced diagonally
1 cup baby spinach leaves
juice of 2 limes
½ cup fresh basil leaves, torn

1. Simmer the stock with the lime leaves, lemon grass, chilli and ginger for about 5 minutes, then add the coconut milk and fish sauce and heat through
2. Add the mushrooms and green beans and simmer gently for about 2–3 minutes
3. Add the prawns and mangetout and continue to simmer for another 3–4 minutes until the prawns have all turned pink and

are just cooked through (do not overcook or the prawns will become tough)
4. Stir through the spring onions, spinach and lime juice and continue to cook until the spinach has just wilted
5. Serve immediately, garnished with fresh basil leaves

THAI-STYLE SPINACH AND WATERCRESS SOUP
Preparation time: 5 minutes
Cooking time: 10–15 minutes

2–3 tbsp olive oil
1 medium brown onion, chopped
3–4 garlic cloves, chopped
½–1 large green chilli, chopped
3–4 fresh lime leaves
1 stalk lemon grass
180g baby spinach leaves
100g mixed watercress, spinach and rocket leaves*
1¼ litres chicken stock, hot
freshly ground black pepper

1. Heat the olive oil, add the onion and sauté for 2–3 minutes, then add the garlic, chilli, lime leaves and lemon grass and continue to sauté for another minute
2. Add the spinach, mixed watercress, spinach and rocket and the hot stock and simmer for about 5–6 minutes
3. Remove the lemon grass and lime leaves, purée the soup and season with black pepper

*Use watercress and/or rocket if a bag of mixed leaves is not available

TOMATO, FENNEL AND SEAFOOD SOUP
Preparation time: 15 minutes
Cooking time: 20 minutes

2–3 tbsp olive oil
1 medium red onion, coarsely chopped
1 medium fennel, coarsely chopped
5–6 garlic cloves, chopped
1 tbsp tomato paste

400g vine-ripened tomatoes, roughly chopped
1 litre vegetable or chicken stock
500g fresh mussels, in their shells
125g raw prawns, peeled
4 baby squid, cut into rings with tentacles separate
125g small scallops
freshly ground black pepper
2 tbsp dill, chopped

1. Heat the olive oil and sauté the onion and fennel for 3–4 minutes, then add the garlic and sauté for another minute
2. Add the tomato paste and tomatoes, stir to coat them in the oil and sauté for 1–2 minutes
3. Add the stock and simmer gently for about 10–15 minutes until the fennel is soft, then purée and strain
4. Reheat the soup to a gentle simmer, add the mussels, cover the pan and cook for 2–3 minutes, then add the prawns and squid tentacles and cook for 2–3 minutes until the mussels have opened and the prawns have just turned pink
5. Add the scallops and squid rings and continue to cook for another minute
6. Season with black pepper and serve garnished with dill

Note: We use fresh, uncooked seafood; if you want to use a precooked seafood mixture, add it to the soup at the end of cooking and heat through for a minute at most, or it will be tough and rubbery

WATERCRESS SOUP
Preparation time: 5 minutes
Cooking time: 15 minutes

1 litre chicken stock
1 heaped tbsp grated fresh ginger
1 green chilli, finely sliced
150g watercress or mixed watercress and baby spinach leaves
4 spring onions, finely sliced
1 tbsp light soya sauce
1 egg (optional)
fresh coriander, chopped

1. Heat the stock with the ginger and chilli and simmer for about 10 minutes
2. Remove the coarse stalks from the watercress and discard, then add the leaves to the soup with the spring onions and simmer gently until the leaves have just wilted (about 1–2 minutes)
3. Take the soup off the heat and stir through the soya sauce
4. Lightly beat the egg then stir it into the soup
5. Serve immediately, garnished with fresh coriander

ZUCCHINI SOUP
Preparation time: 10 minutes
Cooking time: 20–25 minutes

2 tbsp olive oil
1 onion, coarsely chopped
3–4 garlic cloves, sliced
1 green chilli, sliced
1 tbsp ground cumin
1 small potato, peeled and coarsely chopped
600g zucchini, chopped
1 litre chicken stock
freshly ground black pepper
½ cup fresh basil leaves, torn

1. Heat the olive oil and sauté the onion for 2–3 minutes, then add the garlic, chilli and cumin and sauté for another minute
2. Add the potato and zucchini, stir to coat in the oil and continue to sauté for 2–3 minutes
3. Add the stock and simmer gently for 15–20 minutes until the potato is soft, then purée the soup
4. Season with black pepper and serve garnished with basil

SUMPTUOUS SALADS AND SALSAS

VEGETABLE SALADS AND SALSAS

SALADS WITH SEAFOOD

SALADS WITH POULTRY

SALADS WITH MEAT

EGGS

With the fabulous fresh vegetables and fruit around these days, salads no longer have to mean a tasteless assemblage of limp lettuce leaf with chunks of cucumber and tomato and a dollop of bought salad cream. They can be prepared with a minimum of effort and are a great way to include a lot of different ingredients in your diet. Some of these salads are meals in themselves, others are great as an accompaniment to grilled, roast or poached meat or with an omelette or vegetable fritters.

VEGETABLE SALADS AND SALSAS

ASIAN SALAD WITH RICE NOODLES
Preparation time: 10–15 minutes
Cooking time: 5 minutes

1 tbsp olive oil
2 tbsp sesame oil
1 tbsp light soya sauce
1 tbsp fresh lemon juice
1 tbsp sweet chilli sauce
1 tbsp grated fresh ginger
60g dried rice noodles
80g mixed watercress, rocket and spinach leaves
1 red pepper, finely sliced
½ cucumber, diced
4 spring onions, sliced
1 cup mangetout, cut into 3 pieces
50g bamboo shoots
1 cup bean sprouts
1 cup coriander leaves, chopped
½ cup mint leaves, chopped

1. Shake the olive oil, sesame oil, soya sauce, lemon juice, chilli sauce and ginger together and leave to stand for about 15 minutes
2. Cut the rice noodles into 3–4cm lengths and put them into a bowl; pour over boiling water and leave them to soften according to the instructions on the packet, then refresh under cold water, drain and put into a serving bowl

3. Add all the other vegetables and herbs to the noodles and toss to mix everything together

4. Pour over the dressing (there may be a little too much but any left over will keep for a few days in the fridge), toss and serve

Variation: use fresh or dried egg or won ton noodles instead of the rice noodles – just cook according to the instructions on the packet

AVOCADO SALSA
Preparation time: 5 minutes

2 avocados, peeled, stoned and diced
4–5 spring onions, finely sliced
½ cup chopped fresh coriander
2 tbsp lime or lemon juice
freshly ground black pepper

1. Put the avocado into a bowl, add the spring onions and coriander, toss gently with the lemon/lime juice and season with black pepper

BEAN SPROUT AND CUCUMBER SALAD
Preparation time: 6–8 minutes

1 red onion, finely sliced
½ cucumber, seeds removed and diced
4 spring onions, sliced
2 cups bean sprouts
1 red chilli, finely sliced
½ cup fresh coriander leaves, chopped
4 tbsp coconut cream
1 tbsp brown rice vinegar
1 tbsp lemon juice

1. Add the red onion, cucumber, spring onions, bean sprouts, red chilli and coriander leaves to a bowl and gently toss together

2. Shake together the coconut cream, rice vinegar and lemon juice and pour over the salad just before serving

Variation: add a few freshly cooked prawns

CARROT AND BEETROOT SALAD
Preparation time: 15 minutes plus 1 hour to marinate

250g carrots, scrubbed and grated
125g fresh beetroot, peeled and grated
2–3 garlic cloves, crushed
1 cup fresh coriander, chopped
⅓ cup brown rice vinegar

1. Put the carrot, beetroot, garlic and coriander in a salad bowl
2. Pour over the vinegar and toss to mix well
3. Leave to marinate in the fridge for at least an hour (the longer it is left to marinate the tastier it becomes)

CAULIFLOWER SALAD
Preparation time: 5 minutes
Cooking time: 5–6 minutes

1 small cauliflower
4–6 spring onions, finely sliced
1 cup flat-leaf parsley, chopped
⅓ cup olive oil
2 tbsp red-wine vinegar
1 red chilli, finely sliced
freshly ground black pepper

1. Cut the cauliflower into small florets and steam or boil until it is just cooked but still firm (about 5–6 minutes), drain then rinse it under cold water and dry with kitchen paper and put into a serving bowl
2. Add the spring onions and parsley
3. Shake the olive oil, vinegar and chilli together, pour the dressing over the cauliflower, season with black pepper and toss to mix everything together

CITRUS SALAD
Preparation time: 10 minutes

½ cup walnut pieces
1 ruby-red grapefruit
2 navel oranges

1 tbsp walnut oil
1 cup herbed salad leaves
1 chicory, leaves separated
½ cup kalamata olives
½ cup fresh mint leaves, finely chopped
freshly ground black pepper

1. Briefly toast the walnut pieces in a dry frying pan for about a minute, being careful not to burn them
2. Peel and segment the grapefruit and oranges, reserving any juice
3. Shake 2 tablespoons of the reserved fruit juices and the walnut oil together
4. Put the salad leaves, chicory, fruit, olives and mint into a salad bowl, pour over the dressing, season to taste with black pepper and toss to mix well; serve sprinkled with the toasted walnuts

CORN AND CELERY SALSA
Preparation time: 5 minutes
Cooking time: 2–3 minutes

1 cup fresh or frozen sweet corn kernels
1 tbsp olive oil
1 tbsp red-wine vinegar
freshly ground black pepper
2 stalks celery, finely diced
10–12 cherry tomatoes, halved or quartered
1 red onion, finely diced
1 cup flat-leaf parsley, chopped

1. Cook the sweet corn briefly in boiling water, then drain and cool
2. Shake the olive oil, vinegar and black pepper together
3. Put all the ingredients in a salad bowl, pour the dressing over and toss to mix well

CUCUMBER SALAD
Preparation time: 10 minutes
Cooking time: 1–2 minutes

50g peanuts (optional)
1 tsp brown sugar

1 tbsp rice vinegar
1 tsp fish sauce
½ red chilli, finely sliced
¼ cup fresh coriander leaves, chopped
1 long cucumber, peeled, seeded and diced

1. Roast the peanuts, being careful not to burn them, then chop coarsely
2. Dissolve the sugar in the vinegar then stir in the fish sauce
3. Put the chilli, coriander and cucumber in a bowl, pour over the dressing and toss to mix everything together; sprinkle with the chopped peanuts

FENNEL SALAD
Preparation time: 5 minutes

2–3 medium fennel bulbs
1 tbsp small capers
2 tbsp lemon juice
2–3 tbsp olive oil
1 tbsp fennel leaves or tarragon leaves, chopped
freshly ground black pepper
pinch of salt to taste

1. Remove the outer leaves from the fennel, finely slice it vertically (the easiest way is to use a mandolin if you have one), then put it into a salad bowl and add the capers
2. Shake together the lemon juice, olive oil, black pepper and salt, pour over the fennel and toss to mix well

GREEN BEAN SALAD
Preparation time: 5–10 minutes plus 1 ½ hours to marinate
Cooking time: 4–5 minutes

1–2 tbsp red-wine vinegar
2–3 garlic cloves, crushed
2 tbsp chopped flat-leaf parsley
2 tbsp chopped fresh basil
400g green beans
½ red onion, finely sliced
3–4 tbsp olive oil
freshly ground black pepper

1. Mix together the vinegar, garlic, parsley and basil in a serving bowl and leave for at least 30 minutes
2. Steam or boil the green beans until they are just cooked but still crunchy (about 2–3 minutes), drain and add immediately to the dressing, then toss and leave them to marinate for at least an hour
3. Just before serving add the onion and olive oil, toss to mix everything together and season with black pepper

GREEN SALAD
Preparation time: 15–20 minutes

1 small or baby romaine lettuce, coarsely shredded
1 chicory, leaves separated
3–4 stalks celery, finely sliced
1 small green pepper, seeded and diced
16 mangetout, sliced
2 small avocados, peeled, stoned and diced
2 small green apples, cored and diced
1 tbsp fresh lemon juice
fresh flat-leaf parsley, chopped
2 tbsp olive oil
1 tbsp cider vinegar
freshly ground black pepper

1. Prepare all the vegetables, tossing the avocado and apple in a little lemon juice to stop them going brown, and mix them together, with the parsley, in a salad bowl
2. Shake the olive oil, cider vinegar and black pepper together and pour over the salad just before serving

MANGO SALSA
Preparation time: 10 minutes plus 2 hours to marinate

1 mango, peeled and diced
1 small red pepper, cored, seeded and diced
½ red onion or 5–6 spring onions, finely chopped
½–1 red chilli or 5–6 spring onions, finely chopped
½ cup mint leaves, finely chopped
1 cup coriander leaves, finely chopped

2 tbsp fresh lime juice
freshly ground black pepper

1. Put the mango, red pepper, onion, chilli, mint and coriander in a bowl
2. Shake the lime juice and black pepper together, pour over the salsa and toss; allow to stand for 2 hours to let the flavours infuse

Variation: use pineapple instead of the mango

MUSHROOM SALAD
Preparation time: 5 minutes plus 30 minutes to marinate

250g baby mushrooms, cleaned
½ cup flat-leaf parsley, finely chopped
¼ cup olive oil
1 tbsp fresh lemon juice
1 red chilli, finely chopped
1 tsp ground black pepper

1. Put the mushrooms into a serving bowl and gently stir through the parsley, ensuring it is well mixed through
2. Shake the olive oil, lemon juice, chilli and black pepper together, pour over the mushrooms and toss to coat them in the dressing, then leave them to marinate for at least 30 minutes

POTATO AND WATERCRESS SALAD
Preparation time: 10 minutes
Cooking time: 20–25 minutes

500g new potatoes
1 cup watercress leaves
2 stalks celery, finely chopped
4 spring onions, sliced
3–4 tbsp pesto (see page 233)
freshly ground black pepper

1. Steam or boil the potatoes until they are cooked, then drain and put into a serving bowl (cut them in half if they are quite large)

2. Stir through the watercress, celery, spring onions and pesto and season with black pepper

RED PEPPER AND TOMATO SALSA
Preparation time: 5 minutes

2 ripe vine-ripened tomatoes, chopped
1 red pepper, chopped
¾ cup coriander, finely chopped
½ red chilli, finely sliced (optional)
2 tbsp lime or lemon juice
freshly ground black pepper

1. Gently mix together the tomatoes, red pepper, coriander and chilli in a serving bowl
2. Just before serving, stir through the lime juice and season with black pepper

THAI-STYLE GREEN SALAD
Preparation time: 10 minutes

1 tbsp sweet chilli sauce
1 tbsp grated fresh ginger
1 tbsp lemon juice
2 tbsp sesame oil
1 tbsp light soya sauce
100g mixed watercress and rocket
½ cucumber, diced
1 green pepper, diced
1 green apple, diced
1 small red onion, sliced
1 cup bean sprouts
½ cup fresh coriander, chopped
¼ cup fresh mint, chopped

1. Shake the chilli sauce, ginger, lemon juice, sesame oil and soya sauce together
2. Put all the salad ingredients and herbs into a salad bowl, pour over the dressing and serve immediately

TOMATO AND BASIL SALAD
Preparation time: 5 minutes

150g rocket leaves
4 vine-ripened tomatoes, sliced
1 medium red onion, finely sliced
1 cup black olives
½ cup fresh basil leaves, torn
2 tbsp olive oil
1 tbsp balsamic vinegar
freshly ground black pepper

1. Put the rocket, tomatoes, onion, olives and basil in a serving bowl
2. Shake together the olive oil and balsamic vinegar, pour this over the salad and season with black pepper

TOMATO AND CORIANDER SALSA
Preparation time: 10 minutes

3–4 medium vine-ripened tomatoes, chopped
1 small red onion, chopped
6–8 fresh mangetout, coarsely sliced
½ cucumber, chopped
2 spring onions, finely sliced
½ cup fresh coriander leaves, chopped
½ red chilli, finely sliced (optional)
2 tbsp fresh lime juice
freshly ground black pepper

1. Mix all the vegetables, coriander and chilli together in a serving bowl
2. Just before serving, pour over the lime juice and season with black pepper

TOMATO, OLIVE AND ROCKET SALAD
Preparation time: 5 minutes

100g rocket
2 tbsp capers, rinsed and chopped
250g cherry tomatoes, halved

1 cup kalamata olives
4 tbsp olive oil
2 tbsp white-wine vinegar

1. Put the rocket, capers, tomatoes and olives in a bowl
2. Shake the olive oil and vinegar together, pour this over the salad and toss to mix well

ZUCCHINI SALAD
Preparation time: 5 minutes plus 15 minutes to marinate

3–4 small zucchini
2–3 tbsp olive oil
juice of 1 lemon
1 green chilli, finely sliced
½ cup flat-leaf parsley, chopped
freshly ground black pepper

1. Wash and finely slice the zucchini
2. Shake together the olive oil, lemon juice and chilli and pour this over the zucchini
3. Stir through the parsley, season with black pepper and leave for about 15 minutes before serving

SALADS WITH SEAFOOD

CRAB AND APPLE SALAD
Preparation time: 10 minutes

1 Granny Smith apple
1 small fennel bulb
2 tbsp lemon juice
1 cup fresh coriander, chopped
6 spring onions, finely sliced
1 cup bean sprouts
1 220g tin white crab meat in brine, drained
2 tbsp olive oil
1 red chilli, sliced
1 tbsp grated fresh ginger
2–3 cups mixed salad leaves
freshly ground black pepper

1. Core and dice the apple and finely slice the fennel, then put them into a salad bowl and toss with one tablespoon of the lemon juice
2. Add the coriander, spring onions, bean sprouts and crab and toss gently to mix
3. Shake together the olive oil, remaining lemon juice, chilli and ginger and pour over the crab mixture
4. Divide the salad leaves between four plates, top with the crab mixture and season to taste with black pepper

CRAB AND CUCUMBER SALAD
Preparation time: 15 minutes

2 × 170g tins of white crab meat, rinsed and drained
½ cucumber, finely chopped
1 stalk celery, finely sliced
½ fennel bulb, finely chopped
3–4 water chestnuts, finely chopped (optional)
4–6 spring onions, finely sliced
1 red chilli, chopped (or to taste)
2 tsp chopped mint
2 tbsp chopped coriander
2–3 tbsp olive oil
1 tsp Thai fish sauce
2 tbsp lemon juice
2 garlic cloves, crushed
80–100g mixed salad leaves

1. Place the crab meat in a large bowl and break it up with a fork
2. Add the cucumber, celery, fennel, water chestnuts, spring onions, chilli, mint and coriander and mix together well
3. Shake the olive oil, fish sauce, lemon juice and garlic together, pour this over the salad and toss
4. Serve on a bed of mixed salad leaves

Variation: replace half the crab with chopped cooked prawns

GREEN MANGO AND PRAWN SALAD

Preparation time: 15 minutes (plus 30 minutes to chill the dressing)
Cooking time: 2–3 minutes

1 small red chilli, finely sliced, or 1 tsp chilli sambal
1 tbsp fresh lemon juice
2 tbsp fresh lime juice
1 tbsp fish sauce
½ tsp palm or caster sugar
16–20 large raw prawns*
1 large green mango
¼ cup fresh mint leaves, chopped
½ cup fresh coriander leaves
100g mixed watercress, rocket and baby spinach leaves or mixed salad leaves of choice
1 medium red onion
4–5 spring onions, finely chopped
1 cup bean sprouts

1. Shake together the chilli, lemon and lime juices, fish sauce and sugar until the sugar dissolves, then refrigerate for about 30 minutes
2. Cook the prawns in a little boiling water for 2–3 minutes until they have just turned pink – do not overcook – then drain
3. Cut the mango into thin julienne slices (this is most easily done with a mandolin if you have one)
4. Put the mint, coriander, salad leaves, mango, red onion, spring onions, bean sprouts and prawns into a serving bowl, pour over the dressing and mix together well

*You could buy precooked prawns but we think they taste much better if you cook them yourself

SQUID SALAD

Preparation time: 5–10 minutes
Cooking time: 1 minute

1 red chilli, finely sliced
2 tbsp lime juice
2 tbsp Thai fish sauce

½ tsp palm sugar
250g baby squid tubes
2–3 lime leaves, the central rib removed and finely sliced
1 stalk lemon grass, finely chopped
1 cup mixed fresh coriander and mint leaves, finely chopped
1 red onion, finely sliced
1 cup bean sprouts

1. Shake together the red chilli, lime juice, fish sauce and sugar
2. Cut the squid into strips and blanch in boiling water for about
   1 minute, until it has just turned opaque (do not overcook or
   the squid will become tough and rubbery) then drain
3. Toss together the lime leaves, lemon grass, coriander and mint
   leaves, red onion, bean sprouts and squid, pour over the
   dressing and serve immediately

*Variation: Make this salad with prawns instead of squid. Poach
peeled prawns in boiling water briefly for about 1–2 minutes until
they have just turned pink. As with the squid, do not overcook.*

THAI-STYLE CRAB AND MANGO SALAD
Preparation time: 15 minutes

2 cups mixed salad leaves
½ ripe mango, cut into small cubes
1 small avocado, chopped and tossed in lemon juice
½ large red onion, finely sliced
1 cup bean sprouts
½ cup fresh coriander, chopped
¼ cup fresh mint leaves, chopped
170g white crab meat, shredded
1 red chilli, finely chopped
juice of 2 limes
1 tbsp fish sauce
1 tbsp sesame oil

1. Put the salad leaves, mango, avocado, red onion, bean sprouts,
   coriander, mint and the crab in a serving bowl
2. Shake the chilli, lime juice, fish sauce and sesame oil together,
   pour over the salad and toss to mix well

Variation: Make with cooked prawns or poached chicken breast

THAI-STYLE PRAWN AND CITRUS SALAD
Preparation time: 15 minutes
Cooking time: 3 minutes

100g mixed watercress, rocket and spinach leaves
1 red onion, sliced
½ cucumber, julienned
1 cup seedless green grapes, halved
2 small mandarins, peeled and divided into segments
1 cup fresh mint leaves, chopped
1 cup fresh coriander leaves, chopped
2cm strip of fresh ginger, peeled and julienned
1–2 long red chillies, seeded and julienned
3 tbsp olive oil
250g peeled raw tiger prawns
2 tbsp fresh mandarin juice
2 tbsp fresh lemon or lime juice
2 tbsp Thai fish sauce

1. Gently mix together all the salad vegetables, fruit, mint, coriander, ginger and chilli in a salad bowl
2. Heat the olive oil in a frying pan or wok and gently stir-fry the prawns, tossing occasionally for 2–3 minutes until they have all turned pink (do not overcook or they will be tough), then add them to the salad
3. Shake together the mandarin, lemon or lime juice and fish sauce, pour over the salad and toss to mix well

SALADS WITH POULTRY

CHICKEN AND PASTA SALAD
Preparation time: 10 minutes
Cooking time: 10 minutes

1 tsp chilli sambal (or 1 red chilli, chopped)
2 tbsp lemon juice
1 tbsp sesame oil
1 tbsp mirin
1 tbsp soya sauce
2 tsp fish sauce

200g dry pasta such as spiralli or penne
2 chicken breasts, skinned
8 cherry tomatoes, cut into quarters
½ cucumber, diced
½ red or green pepper, seeded and diced
12 mangetout, halved
4–6 spring onions, sliced
1 cup bean sprouts
½ cup fresh coriander, chopped
½ cup fresh mint, chopped

1. Shake the chilli, lemon juice, sesame oil, mirin, soya sauce and fish sauce together
2. Cook the pasta in plenty of boiling water following the instructions on the packet, drain and rinse with cold water
3. Poach the chicken breasts for about 10 minutes or until they are just cooked through, then drain and slice
4. Mix together all the salad ingredients, coriander and mint, add the pasta and chicken, pour over the dressing and toss gently to mix well

MINCED CHICKEN IN LETTUCE LEAVES
Preparation time: 10 minutes
Cooking time: 5 minutes

1–2 iceberg lettuce
2 tbsp peanut oil
2 garlic cloves, finely chopped
2 tbsp grated fresh ginger
8 spring onions, finely sliced
1 red chilli, finely chopped
1 cup frozen peas
8 spring onions, finely sliced
400g minced chicken*
100g water chestnuts, chopped
2 tsp sesame oil
2 tbsp hoisin or oyster sauce
2 tbsp light soya sauce
1 cup fresh coriander leaves, chopped

1. Carefully separate the lettuce leaves, keeping them whole, wash and leave to crisp in iced water, then drain, dry and keep in the fridge
2. Heat the peanut oil, add the garlic, ginger, chilli, spring onions and peas and stir-fry gently for about 1 minute
3. Add the chicken and water chestnuts and continue to stir-fry for another 3–4 minutes until the chicken has all changed colour (do not overcook or the chicken will go tough)
4. Add the sesame oil, hoisin sauce and soya sauce and heat through for another minute, then stir through the fresh coriander
5. Serve the chicken in the lettuce leaves, roll up and eat with your fingers

*If possible mince your own chicken, or get the butcher to mince some chicken thighs for you

ROAST DUCK BREAST WITH BLACK OLIVE AND GRAPEFRUIT SALAD
Preparation time: 10 minutes
Cooking time: 15–20 minutes

3 tbsp olive oil
2–3 duck breasts, skinned
100g mixed watercress, rocket and baby spinach leaves
1 red onion, thinly sliced
200g kalamata olives
1 ruby grapefruit, peeled, divided into segments and halved
6 marinated artichoke hearts, halved
1 tbsp lemon juice
1 tbsp balsamic vinegar
freshly ground black pepper
¼ cup flat-leaf parsley

1. Preheat the oven to 200°C
2. Pour a little of the olive oil over the duck breasts and bake in the oven for about 20 minutes or until they are cooked to your liking, then slice thinly
3. Mix together the mixed spinach, rocket and watercress leaves, onion, olives, grapefruit segments and artichoke hearts

4. Shake the remaining olive oil, lemon juice and balsamic vinegar together, pour over the salad and toss to mix well
5. Divide the salad among the plates, top with the duck slices, season to taste with black pepper and garnish with parsley

THAI-STYLE CHICKEN NOODLE SALAD
Preparation time: 5 minutes
Cooking time: 5 minutes

2 tbsp olive oil
2 chicken breasts, skinned and sliced
100g rice vermicelli noodles
½ cup mixed fresh coriander and mint, finely chopped
2 lime leaves, very finely sliced
4 spring onions, central spine removed and finely sliced
1 cup bean sprouts
12–16 mangetout, sliced
1 tbsp sesame oil
2 tsp fish sauce
1 small red chilli or 1 tsp chilli sambal
juice of 2 limes or 1 lemon

1. Heat the olive oil and stir-fry the chicken until it is thoroughly cooked (about 3–4 minutes)
2. Soak the noodles in boiling water for 2–3 minutes until they are soft (or according to the instructions on the packet) then rinse under cold water and drain
3. Mix together the chicken, mint and coriander, lime leaves, spring onions, bean sprouts, mangetout and noodles
4. Shake together the sesame oil, fish sauce, chilli and lime juice
5. Pour the dressing over the salad, toss and serve immediately

THAI-STYLE MINCED CHICKEN SALAD (LARB)
Preparation time: 15 minutes plus 30 minutes marinating
Cooking time: 5 minutes

1 iceberg or romaine lettuce
½ cucumber
¼ cup chicken stock
1–2 garlic cloves, crushed

¼ tsp palm sugar
250g minced chicken breast or thighs
1 green pepper, finely diced
6 spring onions, sliced
1 red onion, finely sliced
1 cup coriander, chopped
½ cup fresh mint, chopped
1 red chilli or 2 tsp chilli sambal
3 tbsp lime juice
1 tbsp fish sauce

1. Carefully separate the lettuce leaves, wash and crisp in the fridge
2. Cut the cucumber lengthways, remove the seeds and chop finely; put it into a colander, sprinkle with some salt and leave for about 30 minutes, then rinse
3. Heat the stock with the garlic and sugar, add the chicken and simmer, stirring occasionally until it is cooked (about 3–4 minutes)
4. Put the chicken in a serving bowl, add the pepper, cucumber, spring onions, red onion, coriander, mint and chilli
5. Shake together the lime juice and fish sauce, pour over the salad and stir to mix together well
6. Serve spoonfuls of chicken salad into individual lettuce leaves, fold and eat with your fingers

THAI-STYLE CHICKEN SALAD WITH CARROT AND CABBAGE
Preparation time: 10 minutes plus 30 minutes to marinate
Cooking time: 10 minutes

3–4 garlic cloves, crushed
1 tbsp chilli sambal
3 tbsp fresh lime or lemon juice
1 tbsp rice vinegar
2 tsp fish sauce
2 tbsp olive oil
2 tbsp sesame oil
2 chicken breasts, skinned
1 cup green cabbage, grated
1 cup red cabbage, grated

1 cup carrot, grated
½ fennel bulb, grated
1 medium red onion, finely sliced
4–6 spring onions, sliced
1 cup bean sprouts
½ cup fresh mint, chopped
½ cup fresh coriander, chopped

1. Shake the garlic, chilli, lime juice, rice vinegar, fish sauce and oils together and leave for at least half an hour
2. Gently poach the chicken (one method to ensure the chicken is not overcooked is to put the chicken in cold water or stock, bring to a boil, cover, turn off the heat and leave for approximately 20 minutes) or use leftover chicken cut into slices
3. Mix together all the salad ingredients, mint, coriander and chicken, pour over the dressing and toss to mix well

SALADS WITH MEAT

GRILLED LAMB CHOPS WITH MINTED SPINACH SALAD
Preparation time: 10 minutes
Cooking time: 15 minutes

8 small lamb loin chops
1 avocado
1 ½ tbsp lemon juice
150g baby spinach leaves
¼ cantaloupe melon, cut into cubes
½ red pepper, sliced
3–4 spring onions, sliced
1 cup bean sprouts
2 tbsp olive oil
1 tbsp balsamic vinegar
¼ cup chopped fresh mint

1. Grill the lamb chops until cooked to your liking (approximately 15 minutes)
2. Peel, stone and dice the avocado and toss in a little lemon juice
3. Put the avocado, spinach, melon, red pepper, spring onions and bean sprouts into a salad bowl

4. Shake together the olive oil, lemon juice, balsamic vinegar and mint, pour over the salad and toss to mix well
5. Divide the salad between four plates and top with the grilled lamb chops

MINCED PORK IN LETTUCE LEAVES
Preparation time: 15 minutes (if mincing your own pork)
Cooking time: 5 minutes

1 large romaine or iceberg lettuce
1 tbsp vegetable oil
1 tbsp sesame oil
2–3 garlic cloves, chopped
1 tsp chilli sambal
450g pork loin, minced
1 red onion, finely chopped
1 cup fresh coriander, chopped
½ cup mint leaves, chopped
2 tbsp lime or lemon juice
1 tbsp soya sauce

1. Wash the lettuce leaves, dry and put in the fridge to crisp
2. Heat the vegetable and sesame oils and stir-fry the garlic, chilli sambal and minced pork for about 5 minutes until the pork is cooked through
3. Put the onion, coriander and mint in a bowl, add the pork, pour over the lime juice and soya sauce, and toss to mix thoroughly
4. Serve the pork on large lettuce leaves and eat with your fingers

THAI GRILLED VENISON SALAD
Preparation time: 5 minutes
Cooking time: 10–20 minutes plus 10–15 minutes to rest

200g whole piece of venison, sirloin or fillet
1 tsp chilli sambal
3 tbsp lime juice
¼ tsp palm sugar
2 tbsp fish sauce
100g mixed rocket, watercress and spinach leaves
1 large red onion, finely sliced

½ cucumber, seeds removed and julienned
1 red pepper, seeded and finely sliced
4 spring onions, sliced
1 cup coriander, chopped
½ cup mint, chopped

1. Grill the venison to your taste and once cooked set it aside for 10–15 minutes, then slice finely
2. Shake the chilli sambal, lime juice, palm sugar and fish sauce together until the sugar dissolves
3. Mix all the salad ingredients and herbs together, pour over the dressing, toss and serve on individual plates, then top with the venison

EGGS

BEAN FRITTATA
Preparation time: 5 minutes
Cooking time: 10–12 minutes

250g green beans
5 large eggs
1 tbsp water or soya milk
freshly ground black pepper
1 tbsp olive oil
4 garlic cloves, finely chopped
½ green chilli, finely sliced (optional)
5–6 spring onions, finely sliced
1 cup flat-leaf parsley, finely chopped

1. Steam or boil the green beans until they are cooked but still firm, then drain and cut into 2–3 pieces
2. Whisk together the eggs and soya milk and season with black pepper
3. Pour the olive oil into a frying pan and gently fry the garlic, chilli and spring onions for 30 seconds then add the green beans and parsley
4. Pour over the eggs and stir to mix everything together
5. Cook gently for about 3–4 minutes until the eggs are nearly set and the base is firm and slightly browned, then put the pan under a hot grill and cook until the top of the frittata is set

SWEET POTATO FRITTATA
Preparation time: 10 minutes
Cooking time: 15–20 minutes

2–3 large sweet potatoes, peeled
5 large eggs
1 tbsp soya milk
freshly ground black pepper
1 tbsp olive oil
1 large onion, finely sliced
4–5 garlic cloves, finely chopped
½ green chilli, finely sliced
3–4 spring onions, finely sliced
1 cup coriander, chopped

1. Parboil the sweet potatoes until just cooked, then drain, cool slightly and slice thinly
2. Whisk the eggs with the soya milk and season to taste with black pepper
3. Heat the olive oil in a large frying pan and stir-fry the onion for 3–4 minutes then add the garlic, chilli and spring onions and continue to fry for another minute
4. Add the potatoes and cook for another 1–2 minutes, turning them over once or twice until they are heated through, then stir through the coriander
5. Pour over the eggs and stir to mix everything together well
6. Cook gently for about 3–4 minutes until the eggs are nearly set and the base is firm and slightly browned, then put the pan under a hot grill and cook until the top of the frittata is set

We like this served with a little sweet chilli sauce on the side.

SAUCES, DIPS AND SPREADS

BASIL AND PINE NUT PESTO
Preparation time: 5 minutes

2 cups loosely packed fresh basil leaves
2–3 garlic cloves, peeled
½ cup pine nuts
¼–½ cup olive oil

1. Blend all the ingredients together in a food processor to form a paste, adding more oil if necessary

Note: pesto will keep in the fridge for up to a week, but make sure the surface is covered with a thin layer of oil

BLACK OLIVE TAPENADE
Preparation time: 10–15 minutes depending on whether or not you have to stone the olives

2–3 garlic cloves, peeled
⅔ cup fresh flat-leaf parsley
2 tbsp fresh basil leaves
1 tsp black pepper
2 cups olives, stoned (Kalamata olives have the best flavour)
1 tbsp capers
8 anchovy fillets
⅓ cup olive oil

1. Purée all the ingredients to a smooth paste in a food processor, adding a little more olive oil if necessary

Note: can be stored in the fridge for a week

CORIANDER AND MINT DIP
Preparation time: 10 minutes

1–2 large garlic cloves, peeled
2 tbsp grated fresh ginger
1 cup fresh coriander leaves
½ cup fresh mint leaves
1 green chilli
½ red onion
2 tbsp fresh lime juice

½ cucumber, washed, seeds removed and chopped
2 tsp cider vinegar
5 tbsp olive oil
1 tsp brown rice vinegar

1. Blend all the ingredients together until they form a smooth paste

Serve with vegetable crudités, a baked potato or with steamed prawns.

GUACAMOLE
Preparation time: 5 minutes

2 avocados, peeled and chopped
2 tbsp lemon or lime juice
3 spring onions, finely chopped
2 tbsp chopped fresh coriander
1 tsp chopped fresh red chilli

1. Toss the avocado in the lemon juice, add the spring onions, coriander and chilli and stir gently to mix everything together

HUMMUS
Preparation time: 5 minutes (and overnight if using dried chickpeas)
Cooking time: 1–2 hours if using dried chickpeas

1 tin chickpeas (or 175g dried chickpeas soaked overnight and boiled in fresh water for 1–2 hours)
3–4 smallish garlic cloves
⅓ cup tahini
3 tbsp lemon juice
¼–½ cup of water
1 tbsp olive oil
1 tsp paprika

1. Add the chickpeas, garlic, tahini and lemon juice to a food processor or blender and gradually add the water until the hummus reaches a smooth creamy consistency
2. Serve in a shallow bowl with a little olive oil poured on the surface and sprinkled with paprika

MOROCCAN 'ZHOUG' PASTE
Preparation time: 5–10 minutes

2 tsp cumin seeds
8–10 cardamom pods, crushed and seeds removed
80g fresh coriander
20g fresh flat-leaf parsley
3–4 garlic cloves
1 green chilli
1 tsp coarse black pepper
2 tbsp lemon juice
2 tbsp brown rice vinegar
¼ cup olive oil

1. Crush the cumin and cardamom seeds in a pestle and mortar, or grind in a grinding machine
2. Put all the ingredients in a blender or food processor and process to a smooth paste, adding a little more oil if necessary
3. Leave for at least a couple of hours for the flavours to mature

This is a spicy paste that is delicious on toast either by itself or under a grilled mushroom or tomato, or with vegetable crudités.

ROASTED GARLIC AND CANNELLINI BEAN DIP
Preparation time: 10 minutes
Cooking time: 35–40 minutes

1 small garlic head
2 tbsp olive oil
410g tin cannellini beans, rinsed and drained
2–3 tbsp water
2 tbsp chopped chives
1 tsp paprika

1. Preheat the oven to 180°C
2. Slice the top off the garlic head and discard any loose papery skin covering the head, taking care to keep the cloves intact
3. Brush olive oil over the garlic, wrap in foil, and bake in the oven for about 35–40 minutes until the garlic feels soft when squeezed slightly, then cool and remove the skins from the garlic by pinching each clove

4. Add the beans, garlic and olive oil to a food processor or blender and process to a smooth paste, adding water as necessary to make a smooth purée
5. Stir through the chopped chives and sprinkle with paprika

SALSA VERDE
Preparation time: 5–10 minutes

80g fresh flat-leaf parsley
½ cup mint leaves
3–4 garlic cloves
1 green chilli
2 tsp Dijon mustard
1 tsp coarse black pepper
2 tbsp lemon juice
6–8 anchovies
⅓ cup olive oil

1. Put all the ingredients except the oil into a blender or food processor and process, then slowly add the olive oil until you have a thick sauce (add a little more oil if necessary)
2. Leave for at least a couple of hours for the flavours to mature, then store in the fridge

SPICY AUBERGINE PURÉE
Preparation time: 5 minutes
Cooking time: 35 minutes

1 large aubergine
1 tbsp lemon juice
3 tbsp olive oil
1 small onion, chopped
3–4 garlic cloves, crushed
1 tbsp ginger, grated
1 tsp cumin powder
½ tsp cayenne pepper
4 spring onions, finely sliced
1 tbsp lemon juice
freshly ground black pepper
½ cup fresh coriander and/or mint, chopped

1. Preheat the oven to 220°C
2. Roast the aubergine for about 30 minutes or until soft, cool, peel and purée with the lemon juice in a food processor
3. Heat the olive oil and fry the onion for 3–4 minutes, then add the garlic, ginger, cumin and cayenne pepper and continue to sauté for another minute
4. Add the puréed aubergine and sauté for a further two minutes
5. Stir through the spring onions and lemon juice, season to taste and serve garnished with the coriander and/or mint

THAI GREEN CURRY PASTE
Preparation time: 10–15 minutes

2–3 green chillies (or more to taste), sliced
3–4 garlic cloves, peeled
1 tbsp grated fresh ginger (or galangal if you can find it)
2 tsp ground coriander
1 tsp ground cumin
½ tsp turmeric
1 tsp coarse black pepper
1 cup fresh coriander, including stems, leaves and roots, well washed
1 small red onion, peeled and coarsely chopped
1 tbsp lemon or lime zest
2 tbsp olive oil
1 tsp shrimp paste

1. Put all the ingredients into a blender and process to a smooth paste; add a little water if necessary

It should keep for a month in the fridge, but ensure the top is covered with a thin layer of olive oil.

This is used as a base for green curry vegetables (page 243) or chicken and can also be used as a marinade.

THAI RED CURRY PASTE
Preparation time: 15–20 minutes

3–4 red chillies, sliced
4–5 garlic cloves, peeled

1 tbsp grated fresh ginger or galangal or 3 tsp powdered galangal
1 stalk lemon grass, white part only
4 lime leaves, centre rib removed
1 tsp ground cumin
1 tsp ground coriander
1 tsp coarse black pepper
2 tsp paprika
1 tsp turmeric
1 tbsp coriander roots (optional)
1 small red onion, coarsely chopped
2 tsp lemon or lime zest
2 tbsp olive oil
2 tsp shrimp paste

1. Put all the ingredients into a blender and process to a smooth paste, adding a little water if necessary

This can be stored in the fridge for up to a month.

This sauce is used as a base for chicken, prawn or vegetable curries and is excellent as a marinade (see pages 243, 282 and 319).

TOMATO SAUCE
Preparation time: 5 minutes
Cooking time: 30 minutes

2 tbsp olive oil
1 red onion, chopped
3–4 garlic cloves, chopped
1 red chilli
5–6 sage leaves
1 bay leaf
150g tomato paste
500g ripe vine-ripened tomatoes, chopped
freshly ground black pepper
½ cup fresh basil leaves, chopped

1. Heat the olive oil and sauté the onion for 3–4 minutes until it is translucent

2. Add the garlic, chilli, sage and bay leaves and sauté for another minute, then add the tomato paste, stir and continue to sauté until it turns colour
3. Add the tomatoes, season with black pepper, cover and simmer for about 20 minutes, stirring occasionally
4. Add the chopped basil just before serving

This sauce is excellent with pasta or as a sauce with pizza or with gnocchi.

WALNUT AND PARSLEY PESTO
Preparation time: 5 minutes

2 cups flat-leaf parsley
2–3 garlic cloves, peeled
¼–½ cup olive oil
1 tbsp lemon juice
½ cup walnuts

1. Blend all the ingredients together in a food processor to form a smooth paste, adding more oil if necessary

Note: pesto will keep in the fridge for up to a week, but make sure the surface is covered with a layer of olive oil

Meals to Live For

GUIDELINES

- *Less than 25 per cent of the entire meal should comprise animal protein*
- *Lightly cooked vegetables*
- *Thoroughly cooked meats and fish*
- *Mostly fruit for dessert*

VITAL VEGETABLES

Many of the vegetable dishes are stir-fried. This traditional Chinese way of cooking ensures that vegetables are cooked for a minimum and retain their crunchy character and bright colour. The vegetables are sealed in a little oil, then a little stock, water or other flavouring is added and the vegetables heated through, while stirring. This does not result in 'fried' vegetables as we know them in the West. It is important that the wok is heated before adding the oil so the oil does not burn.

Many of these vegetable dishes are meals in themselves, but others are best as either accompaniments to other dishes or at least served with steamed rice or noodles.

CHINESE BROCCOLI IN OYSTER SAUCE
Preparation time: 5–10 minutes
Cooking time: 5 minutes

1 tbsp olive oil
3 garlic cloves, finely chopped
1 tbsp grated fresh ginger
1 tsp sweet chilli sauce
4 spring onions, finely chopped
500g Chinese broccoli or choi sum, cut into 3cm lengths
1 tbsp light soya sauce
1 tbsp Chinese rice wine
2 tbsp oyster sauce
½ tbsp sesame oil
½ cup chicken stock or water

1. Heat the wok, add the oil and heat for about 30 seconds, then add the garlic, ginger, chilli and spring onions and stir-fry for 1 minute
2. Add the Chinese broccoli, stir to coat in the oil, then add the soya sauce, rice wine, oyster sauce, sesame oil and stock or water, cover and cook briskly for another 2–3 minutes until the broccoli is just tender

GNOCCHI WITH PESTO AND GREEN BEANS

Although it sounds like a lot of effort to make your own gnocchi, it is not actually that difficult (the second time is much easier!).

Preparation time: 30–40 minutes
Cooking time: 20–25 minutes

500g boiling potatoes
½–1 cup flour
200g green beans, topped, tailed and halved
2 tbsp pesto (page 233)

1. Boil the whole potatoes in their skins until they are cooked (do not cut into pieces or prick with a fork as they will absorb water and will be difficult to manage), then drain, peel and mash
2. Slowly add the flour and knead into a smooth paste – it should be soft and smooth but still sticky
3. Dust your worktop or board with flour and roll the potato paste into a sausage-like roll about 2½cm thick, then cut into 1cm pieces
4. Add the gnocchi in batches to a large pan of boiling water and remove about 10 seconds after they have floated to the surface – you will need to test because the cooking time will vary slightly depending on the consistency – and keep warm
5. Steam or boil the green beans for 2–3 minutes until cooked but still crispy
6. Divide the gnocchi, beans and pesto among four soup bowls and toss to mix

Note: If the gnocchi collapse during cooking, the potatoes are too wet and you will need to add an egg to the remaining paste and remix.

GREEN BEANS WITH GINGER

Preparation time: 2 minutes
Cooking time: 6–8 minutes

2 tbsp olive oil
450g green beans, topped and tailed
1 tbsp grated fresh ginger
½ tsp chilli sambal

1. Heat the olive oil, add the beans and sauté for 3–4 minutes
2. Add the ginger and chilli sambal and continue to sauté for another 2–3 minutes or until the beans are cooked but still crisp

GREEN CURRY VEGETABLES
Preparation time: 15 minutes
Cooking time: 10 minutes

3 tbsp green curry paste (page 237)
4–5 lime leaves
400ml coconut milk
½ aubergine, diced
1 green pepper, sliced
1 cup green beans, sliced
½ cup baby mushrooms
1 tbsp fish sauce
½ cup mangetout
½ cup bamboo shoots
½ cup baby sweet corn
½ cup fresh basil
½ cup fresh coriander
2 tbsp lemon juice
1 cup bean sprouts

1. Fry the green curry paste with the lime leaves in a large saucepan for 1 minute, then add the coconut milk and heat through, stirring to mix through the curry paste – do not boil
2. Add the aubergine, green pepper, beans, mushrooms and fish sauce and simmer for 3–4 minutes, then add the mangetout, bamboo shoots and baby sweet corn and continue to simmer for 2–3 minutes until all the vegetables are cooked
3. Stir through the basil, coriander, lemon juice and bean sprouts and serve immediately with steamed rice

Variation: Add diced chicken, prawns or firm bean curd

GRILLED VEGETABLES
Choose any selection of your favourite vegetables to make a delicious, healthy starter or to accompany grilled or baked fish or

meat. The following is a selection we like, but select the vegetables you like or have to hand.

Preparation time: 10 minutes
Cooking time: 5–10 minutes if grilling or 30–40 minutes if roasting

8–12 garlic cloves, peeled (optional)
½ red pepper, seeded and sliced
½ green pepper, seeded and sliced
4 field mushrooms, peeled
1 small fennel bulb, sliced horizontally
4 vine tomatoes, halved, or 8 cherry tomatoes
2 chicory, cut in half
4 pieces asparagus, cut into 2½cm lengths
1 small fresh sweet corn cob, cut into 4, or 12–16 baby sweet corn
2–3 tbsp olive oil

1. Toss all the vegetables in the olive oil and grill or roast them until they are cooked.

Note: Grilling makes vegetables crisper than roasting and takes much less time. If vegetables are roasted, it is better to cook the mushrooms in a separate pan.

MUSHROOM AND PEA CURRY
Preparation time: 10 minutes
Cooking time: 6–8 minutes

3 tbsp olive oil
2–3 garlic cloves, sliced
1½ tsp madras curry powder
½ tsp turmeric
½ tsp cayenne pepper
200g baby mushrooms
1 cup fresh or frozen peas
1 cup fresh or frozen sweet corn kernels
3–4 medium vine-ripened tomatoes, chopped
6–8 spring onions, coarsely sliced
½ cup soya yoghurt or coconut milk
1 tsp garam masala
½ cup fresh coriander

1. Heat the olive oil and stir-fry the garlic, curry powder, turmeric and cayenne pepper for about a minute
2. Add the mushrooms and fresh peas and sweet corn and stir-fry for another minute, then add the tomatoes and simmer for about 5–6 minutes
3. If using frozen peas and sweet corn add them at this stage and heat through
4. Stir through the spring onions, add the soya yoghurt or coconut milk and heat through, but do not boil
5. Serve sprinkled with garam masala and garnish with coriander

NEW POTATOES WITH GREEN BEANS AND PESTO
Preparation time: 2 minutes
Cooking time: 20–25 minutes

8–12 new potatoes
250g green beans
80g mangetout
1 cup rocket leaves
2 tbsp pesto (page 233)

1. Separately steam or boil the potatoes (20–25 minutes), beans (3–4 minutes) and mangetout (1–2 minutes) until cooked, then drain, put into a bowl and stir through the rocket and pesto

PAPRIKA POTATOES
Preparation time: 5–10 minutes
Cooking time: 30 minutes

2–3 large potatoes, washed and scrubbed
2 tbsp olive oil
1 medium onion, finely chopped
2–3 garlic cloves, sliced
1 tbsp paprika
2–3 tbsp finely chopped flat-leaf parsley

1. Boil or steam the potatoes until they are just cooked, then drain, cool slightly and cut into cubes
2. Heat the olive oil and fry the onion for 3–4 minutes, then add the garlic and continue to fry for another minute

3. Add the potato, sprinkle over the paprika and toss to coat the potatoes in the oil
4. Fry the potatoes until they are brown and crisp on the outside, drain on kitchen paper then toss with the parsley

POTATO AND SWEET CORN CURRY
Preparation time: 15 minutes
Cooking time: 15–20 minutes

600g new potatoes
2–3 tbsp olive oil
1 tsp cumin seeds
1 small onion, sliced
2–3 garlic cloves, sliced
½ long green chilli, sliced
1 tbsp ground cumin
1 tsp turmeric
1 tsp cayenne pepper
6 spring onions, finely sliced
2 cups frozen sweet corn kernels
2 cups baby spinach leaves
1 cup fresh coriander, chopped
1 tbsp lemon juice

1. Boil or steam the potatoes until they are just cooked, drain, cool and cut into cubes
2. Heat the olive oil in a large saucepan or wok and fry the cumin seeds for about 30 seconds, then add the onion and fry for 2–3 minutes until it is soft and translucent
3. Add the garlic, chilli, cumin, turmeric and cayenne pepper and cook for another minute
4. Add the potatoes and a little water in the pan, stir to coat in the spices and cook for about 5 minutes until they are heated through, then add the spring onions and sweet corn, and continue to cook until heated through, stirring occasionally to stop them burning
5. Add the spinach and cook for about a minute until it has just wilted, then stir through the coriander and lemon juice

RATATOUILLE
Preparation time: 15 minutes
Cooking time: 35–40 minutes

3 tbsp olive oil
1 large red onion, thinly sliced
3–4 garlic cloves, sliced
1 tsp cumin seeds
1 tsp ground coriander
1 tbsp tomato paste
1 medium aubergine, diced
1 red pepper, seeded and diced
1 yellow or orange pepper, seeded and diced
2 small zucchini, diced
4 vine-ripened tomatoes, quartered
freshly ground black pepper
½ cup fresh flat-leaf parsley, chopped

1. Heat the olive oil and sauté the onion for 3–4 minutes until translucent
2. Add the garlic, cumin seeds and ground coriander and sauté for another minute, then add the tomato paste, aubergine and peppers, cover the pan and cook gently for about 15 minutes
3. Add the zucchini and tomatoes, season with black pepper, cover the pan and continue to cook for another 15 minutes
4. Just before serving stir through the chopped parsley

Note: If you prefer you can roast the vegetables, coated in olive oil, for about 35–40 minutes

ROAST MUSHROOMS
Preparation time: 5 minutes
Cooking time: 15–20 minutes

8 medium to large flat mushrooms
2 tbsp olive oil
1 tbsp balsamic vinegar
a few rocket leaves
freshly ground black pepper
cup flat-leaf parsley, finely chopped

1. Preheat the oven to 200°C
2. Peel the mushrooms and remove the stalk if it is long, then put them into a baking dish
3. Shake the olive oil and vinegar together and pour over the mushrooms
4. Bake for about 20 minutes until cooked
5. Serve on a bed of rocket leaves, season with black pepper and garnish with the chopped parsley

SAUTÉED CAULIFLOWER WITH TOMATOES AND CAPERS
Preparation time: 5–6 minutes
Cooking time: 30 minutes

1 small or medium cauliflower cut into small florets
2–3 tbsp olive oil
2–3 garlic cloves, sliced
1 red chilli, sliced
2–3 heaped tbsp small capers
12–16 cherry tomatoes
5–6 spring onions, sliced
freshly ground black pepper
1 cup fresh flat-leaf parsley, chopped

1. Steam or boil the cauliflower until cooked but still crisp
2. Heat the olive oil in a wok, add the garlic, chilli and capers and sauté for about a minute
3. Add the cooked cauliflower and tomatoes, then sauté until the tomatoes are just cooked through and their skins are beginning to burst
4. Add the spring onions, season with black pepper and continue to sauté for another minute, then stir through the parsley

SAUTÉED MUSHROOMS
Preparation time: 5–6 minutes
Cooking time: 5–6 minutes

4 large portabella mushrooms
2 tbsp olive oil
2 garlic cloves, chopped
½ cup dry white wine or chicken stock

1 tsp ground black pepper
½ cup flat-leaf parsley, chopped

1. Peel and slice the mushrooms
2. Heat the olive oil and briefly sauté the garlic, then add the mushrooms, stir to coat in the oil and sauté for 2–3 minutes
3. Add the wine or stock and sauté briskly for another 2–3 minutes until the mushrooms are cooked
4. Season with black pepper and carefully stir through the parsley

SAUTÉED PEPPERS AND TOMATOES
These are delicious served on toast or with grilled fish or chicken.

Preparation time: 10 minutes
Cooking time: 25–30 minutes

2 tbsp olive oil
1 large red onion, sliced
3–4 garlic cloves, sliced
3 red peppers*, seeded and sliced
4 medium vine-ripened tomatoes, sliced
freshly ground black pepper
1 tbsp balsamic vinegar

1. Heat the olive oil in a large frying pan and sauté the onion for 3–4 minutes, then add the garlic and sauté for another minute
2. Add the peppers, stir to coat in the oil, cover the pan and cook for about 10 minutes
3. Add the tomatoes, season with black pepper, and continue to cook for another 10 minutes
4. Add the balsamic vinegar and continue to cook for another 1–2 minutes

These are delicious served on toast or with grilled fish or chicken.

*A mixture of red, orange and yellow peppers is an attractive alternative to just red peppers

SPICY FRIED SWEET POTATOES
Preparation time: 5 minutes
Cooking time: 30 minutes

2–3 medium to large sweet potatoes, peeled and cut into large pieces

2–3 tbsp olive oil
1 tbsp ground cumin
1 tsp cayenne pepper

1. Steam or boil the sweet potatoes until they are just cooked (about 15 minutes), then drain, allow to cool slightly and dice
2. Heat the oil, add the spices and fry for about 1 minute, then add the potato and stir to coat it in the oil
3. Fry, turning occasionally, until the potatoes are browned and crisp on the outside

These can also be cooked under the grill or roasted in the oven rather than fried.

Variation: use ordinary potatoes

SPICY MASHED SWEET POTATOES
Preparation time: 5 minutes
Cooking time: 20–25 minutes

400g sweet potatoes, peeled and diced
1 tbsp fresh lemon juice
2–3 tbsp olive oil
½ tsp mustard seeds
1 onion, chopped
4–5 garlic cloves, crushed
1 red chilli, sliced
½ tsp turmeric
½ tsp ground cumin
½ tsp ground coriander
½ tsp cayenne pepper

1. Boil the potatoes for about 15 minutes in a large pan until they are cooked, then mash them with the lemon juice and 2 tablespoons of the olive oil and keep warm
2. Heat the remaining olive oil in a frying pan and fry the mustard seeds for 1 minute, then add the onion and sauté for 3–4 minutes
3. Add the garlic, chilli and spices and continue to fry for another minute
4. Stir the onion and spices into the potato ensuring they are well mixed through

SPINACH WITH SESAME SEEDS
Preparation time: 5 minutes
Cooking time: 5 minutes

1 tsp sesame seeds
1 tbsp olive oil
2 garlic cloves, crushed
4 spring onions, sliced
zest of one lemon
180g baby spinach leaves
1 tbsp balsamic vinegar

1. Lightly toast the sesame seeds in a small frying pan for 1–2 minutes – do not overcook – then remove them from the pan
2. Heat the olive oil in a sauté pan and stir-fry the garlic, spring onions and lemon zest for about a minute
3. Add the spinach, stirring to coat it in the oil, cover and cook, stirring occasionally to mix up the spinach for 2–3 minutes until the spinach has just wilted
4. Remove from the heat, pour over the balsamic vinegar and toss to coat the spinach
5. Serve sprinkled with the sesame seeds

STIR-FRIED BOK CHOY
Preparation time: 5 minutes
Cooking time: 5 minutes

400g bok choy
2 tbsp olive oil
2–3 garlic cloves, crushed
1 tbsp grated fresh ginger
3 tbsp water or stock
1 tbsp light soya sauce
1 tsp sesame oil

1. Cut the root off the bok choy and cut it in half or into quarters
2. Heat the oil in a wok and stir-fry the garlic and ginger briefly, then add the bok choy, stock and soya sauce, cover and simmer for 2–3 minutes until the bok choy is tender
3. Toss with the sesame oil and serve immediately

STIR-FRIED SPINACH WITH BEAN SPROUTS
Preparation time: 1 minute
Cooking time: 2-3 minutes

2 tbsp olive oil
2–3 garlic cloves, crushed
6 spring onions, sliced
180g baby spinach leaves
100g bean sprouts
1 tbsp soya sauce

1. Heat the olive oil and sauté the garlic and spring onions for about a minute
2. Add the spinach, bean sprouts and soya sauce and continue to sauté for another minute or until the spinach has just wilted

TOMATO TART
This looks complicated but is actually very easy and absolutely delicious

Preparation time: 5 minutes plus 30 minutes for pastry to cool
Cooking time: 30–35 minutes

1 sheet bought non-dairy puff pastry, defrosted*
1 egg white (to brush the pastry)
3–4 tbsp olive oil
1 large red onion, finely chopped
3–4 garlic cloves, chopped
3–4 large vine-ripened tomatoes, sliced
fresh basil leaves, shredded
freshly ground black pepper

1. Cut the pastry into a large round; place into a greased baking tray or tart pan and put into the fridge for about 30 minutes
2. Preheat the oven to 220°C
3. Brush the pastry with the egg white, prick it all over and bake for about 10 minutes until it has puffed up and is a golden-brown colour, then take it out of the oven, turn it over and brush the other side with the remaining egg white; return it to the oven for 5–6 minutes until the top has become crispy and brown

4. In the meantime, heat 1–2 tablespoons of the olive oil and sauté the onion for 3–4 minutes until it is soft and translucent; add the garlic and continue to sauté for another minute, then remove from the heat and cool

5. Spread the onion mixture evenly over the cooked pastry, arrange the tomato slices in overlapping circles on top of the onions, brush with the remaining olive oil and season with black pepper to taste (the tart can be prepared to this stage and left out of the fridge until just before you are nearly ready to eat)

6. Put the tart into the oven and bake for 15–20 minutes, then serve garnished with the shredded basil

*Non-dairy puff pastry is readily available in supermarkets

VEGETABLE CURRY
Preparation time: 10–15 minutes
Cooking time: 25–30 minutes

3 tbsp olive oil
1 tsp mustard seeds
1 large onion, coarsely chopped
4 garlic cloves, chopped
2 tbsp grated fresh ginger
1 red chilli, sliced
1 tsp cayenne powder
1 tbsp ground cumin
2 tsp ground coriander
1 tsp turmeric
½ small cauliflower, cut into small florets
2 medium potatoes, scrubbed and diced
1–1 ½ cups water
2 large tomatoes chopped
1 small zucchini, sliced
6–8 small mushrooms, halved
1 cup fresh or frozen peas
1 cup fresh or frozen sweet corn kernels
1 cup fresh coriander leaves, chopped

1. Heat the oil in a wok and fry the mustard seeds for about a minute or until they start popping, then add the onion and stir-fry for 2–3 minutes

2. Add the garlic, ginger, chilli and dry spices and stir-fry for a minute before adding the cauliflower and potato, stir to coat them with the spices, then add the water, cover the pan and simmer briskly for about 10–15 minutes
3. Add the tomatoes, zucchini, mushrooms and fresh peas and sweet corn, and continue to simmer for another 5 minutes or until all the vegetables are tender (if using frozen peas and sweet corn, add them after 3–4 minutes and continue to cook until they are heated through)
4. Stir through the fresh coriander leaves

ZUCCHINI AND TOMATO CURRY
Preparation time: 10 minutes
Cooking time: 10 minutes

3 tbsp olive oil
1 tsp cumin seeds
1 small onion, sliced
2–3 garlic cloves, sliced
1 tbsp grated fresh ginger
1 green chilli (optional)
1 tsp ground cumin
1 tsp cayenne pepper
½ tsp turmeric
1 large vine-ripened tomato, chopped
2–3 medium zucchini, sliced and cut into quarters
1 cup frozen peas
1 cup fresh coriander, chopped
1 tbsp lemon juice

1. Heat the olive oil and briefly fry the cumin seeds until they just change colour, then add the onion and fry for 2–3 minutes until it becomes transparent
2. Add the garlic, ginger and chilli, ground cumin, cayenne pepper and turmeric, stir and cook for another minute
3. Add the tomato and continue to fry for another 1–2 minutes, then add the zucchini, stir to coat in the spices and leave to simmer gently, stirring occasionally; add the peas and continue to cook until the peas are heated through (add a little water if necessary)
4. Remove from the heat and stir through the coriander and lemon juice

GREAT GRAINS

COUSCOUS

NOODLES AND PASTA

RICE

Grains, including couscous, noodles, pasta and rice, together with nuts, soya and other legumes are the most important source of protein in vegan diets.

COUSCOUS

COUSCOUS WITH ASPARAGUS AND PEAS
Preparation time: 5 minutes
Cooking time: 6 minutes

2 ½ cups vegetable or chicken stock
2 cups couscous
2 tbsp olive oil
3–4 garlic cloves, crushed
8 stalks asparagus, cut into 4 pieces
16 mangetout, halved
4 spring onions, sliced
1 cup frozen peas
freshly ground black pepper
1 tbsp sesame seeds
fresh basil leaves, torn

1. Heat the stock, pour it over the couscous and leave to stand for about 5–6 minutes or according to the instructions on the packet
2. Heat the olive oil and sauté the garlic and asparagus for about 1 minute, add a little water, cover and cook for another 3 minutes (if using fresh peas, add to the olive oil about three minutes before the asparagus)
3. Add the mangetout, spring onions and frozen peas, and continue to cook for another 1–2 minutes until the peas are warmed through
4. Stir the vegetables through the couscous
5. Season with pepper and serve sprinkled with sesame seeds and basil leaves

COUSCOUS WITH SALMON AND CUCUMBER
We recommend salmon with the bones as they are good for your calcium intake.

Preparation time: 5 minutes
Cooking time: 5–6 minutes

2 ½ cups vegetable or chicken stock, or hot water
2 cups couscous
400g tinned red salmon with bones, drained
1 cucumber, finely chopped
2 tomatoes, finely chopped
1 small red onion, finely chopped
1 cup fresh parsley, chopped
freshly ground black pepper
3 tbsp olive oil
2 tbsp lemon juice
1–2 cups mixed salad leaves

1. Pour the hot stock over the couscous, cover and leave to stand for 5–6 minutes
2. Break up the salmon and the bones with a fork, removing any large bits of skin
3. Add the salmon, cucumber, tomatoes, onion and parsley to the couscous, mix well and season with black pepper
4. Shake the oil and lemon juice together and pour over the couscous
5. Serve on a bed of mixed salad leaves

COUSCOUS WITH TOMATO AND PEPPERS
Preparation time: 10 minutes
Cooking time: 5–6 minutes

2 cups couscous
2 cups vegetable or chicken stock
1 green pepper, seeded and finely diced
4 medium vine-ripened tomatoes, diced
1 red onion, finely diced
1 cup rocket leaves
1 cup flat-leaf parsley, finely chopped
¼ cup fresh mint leaves, chopped

freshly ground black pepper
4 tbsp olive oil
2 tbsp lemon juice

1. Put the couscous in a bowl, pour over the stock, stir and then cover and leave for 5–6 minutes until the stock is absorbed, then leave to cool
2. Just before serving, stir through all the vegetables and herbs and season with black pepper
3. Shake the olive oil and lemon juice together and stir through the couscous

COUSCOUS WITH TOMATO AND WALNUTS
Preparation time: 10 minutes plus 1 hour to marinate

6 medium vine-ripened tomatoes or a 400g tinned tomatoes
1 garlic clove
1 tsp tomato paste
2 tbsp lemon juice
1 cup couscous
3 tbsp olive oil
1 tsp chilli sambal
1 small red onion, finely diced
¼ cup walnut pieces
¼ cup pistachio nuts
½ cup flat-leaf parsley, finely chopped
freshly ground black pepper

1. Purée the tomatoes with the garlic, tomato paste and lemon juice, pour over the couscous and leave for about an hour until the liquid has been absorbed
2. Stir through the olive oil, chilli sambal, red onion, nuts and parsley and season with black pepper

NOODLES AND PASTA

FETTUCCINE WITH TOMATO, OLIVES AND BASIL
Preparation time: 5 minutes
Cooking time: 10–15 minutes

400g fettuccine
2 tbsp olive oil

1 red onion, chopped
3–4 garlic cloves, finely sliced
1 red chilli, sliced
400g tomatoes, chopped
¼ cup black olives
½ cup basil leaves, shredded
freshly ground black pepper

1. Cook the pasta in plenty of boiling water according to the instructions on the packet
2. While the pasta is cooking, heat the olive oil and sauté the onion for 2–3 minutes, then add the garlic and chilli and continue to sauté for another minute
3. Add the tomatoes and simmer for 4–5 minutes, then stir through the olives and basil and season to taste with black pepper
4. Divide the pasta between four plates and top with the sauce

FRESH NOODLES WITH STIR-FRIED PRAWNS AND BROCCOLI
Preparation time: 10 minutes
Cooking time: 12–15 minutes

250g egg noodles
2 tbsp olive oil
3–4 garlic cloves, crushed
1 tbsp fresh ginger, grated
1 long green chilli, chopped
200g broccoli, cut into small florets
½ cup vegetable or chicken stock
300g raw prawns
16 baby mushrooms
220g tinned bamboo shoots or water chestnuts
60g mangetout
1 tbsp oyster sauce
fresh coriander

1. Cook the noodles in plenty of boiling water according to the instructions on the packet, drain and keep warm
2. Heat the olive oil and stir-fry the garlic, ginger and chilli for 1 minute

3. Add the broccoli, stir to ensure it is coated in the oil, then add the stock, cover and simmer for 3–4 minutes
4. Add the prawns and mushrooms and continue to cook for a further 3–4 minutes until all the prawns are pink
5. Add the bamboo shoots, mangetout and oyster sauce and cook for another 2 minutes
6. Divide the noodles between four dishes, top with the prawns and vegetables and garnish with coriander

Variation: use scallops or mixed seafood instead of prawns

LINGUINE WITH ROAST CHERRY TOMATOES AND MANGETOUT
Preparation time: 5 minutes
Cooking time: 30–35 minutes

400g cherry tomatoes
5 tbsp olive oil
2 tbsp balsamic vinegar
400g linguine
300g mangetout, trimmed
3–4 garlic cloves, finely sliced
8 spring onions, finely sliced
6–8 anchovy fillets, chopped
½ cup chopped coriander, basil or flat-leaf parsley

1. Preheat the oven to 160°C
2. Place the tomatoes in a baking tray, sprinkle with 2 tablespoons of the olive oil and the balsamic vinegar and bake for about 30 minutes until soft and slightly dried
3. Bring a saucepan of water to a rolling boil, add the pasta and cook according to the instructions on the packet
4. Pour boiling water over the mangetout and blanch for about 2 minutes, then drain and halve
5. Just before the pasta is finished cooking, heat the remaining olive oil in a saucepan, add the garlic, spring onions and anchovies and cook for about 1 minute, add the mangetout and herbs and continue to cook for another minute, then stir through the tomatoes and any remaining liquid
6. Drain the pasta and divide between four bowls, top with the sauce and toss

LINGUINE WITH ZUCCHINI AND SPINACH
Preparation time: 10 minutes
Cooking time: 10–15 minutes

3–4 garlic cloves
½ green chilli
2 cups fresh basil leaves
½ cup or 100g pine nuts or walnuts
¼–½ cup olive oil plus 1 tbsp extra
450g dried linguine
4 medium zucchini, finely chopped
6 spring onions, sliced
180g baby spinach leaves
2 tbsp lemon juice
freshly ground black pepper

1. In food processor or blender, process the garlic, chilli, basil leaves, pine nuts/walnuts and ¼ cup olive oil, adding more olive oil if necessary until it forms a 'runny' pesto
2. Cook the linguine in plenty of boiling water according to the instructions on the packet, then drain and keep warm if necessary
3. Heat 1 tablespoon of the olive oil in a frying pan or wok, add the zucchini and sauté for 3–4 minutes until it has become soft
4. Add the spring onions and spinach and continue to sauté until the spinach has just wilted, then stir through the lemon juice and 2 tablespoons of the pesto and sauté for another minute until it has heated through
5. Divide the linguine between 4 plates, top with the zucchini and season with black pepper

The remaining pesto will keep in the fridge for at least a week as long as it has a layer of olive oil on the surface.

PASTA WITH PRAWNS AND PEAS
Preparation time: 5 minutes
Cooking time: 10 minutes

400g penne
3 tbsp olive oil
3–4 garlic cloves, crushed

1 green chilli, chopped
½ cup dry white wine or vegetable stock
250g prawns, peeled
1 cup frozen peas
100g mangetout
4–5 spring onions, sliced
1 tbsp lemon juice
½ cup fresh coriander or Italian parsley, coarsely chopped
freshly ground black pepper

1. Cook the pasta in plenty of boiling water following the instructions on the packet and drain
2. While the pasta is cooking, heat the olive oil in a wok or sauté pan and stir-fry the garlic and chilli for about 10 seconds, then add the wine or stock and simmer for 5 minutes
3. Add the prawns and continue to simmer until they turn pink
4. Add the peas, mangetout and spring onions and cook for a further 1–2 minutes
5. Stir through the lemon juice, coriander or parsley, season with black pepper and sauté for another minute
6. Divide the pasta among four serving plates and top with the prawn sauce

PENNE WITH ASPARAGUS AND RED PEPPER
Preparation time: 10 minutes
Cooking time: 15 minutes

400g penne
2 tbsp olive oil
1 cup basil or sage leaves
1 onion, finely sliced
2–3 garlic cloves
1 red chilli, finely chopped (optional)
1 red pepper, seeded and sliced
1 cup fresh or frozen peas
12–16 thin asparagus spears, sliced
½ cup vegetable or chicken stock
freshly ground black pepper

1. Bring a large saucepan of water to a rolling boil, add the penne and cook according to the instructions on the packet, then drain
2. While the penne is cooking, heat the olive oil in a frying pan and fry the basil or sage leaves until they are crisp, then remove them and drain on kitchen paper
3. Add the onion to the oil and sauté for 3–4 minutes; add the garlic and chilli and sauté for another minute; add the pepper and peas and cook for a further 2–3 minutes, then finally add the asparagus and stock, cover and cook for 2–3 minutes until the asparagus is just cooked.
4. Put the penne into a serving dish, top with asparagus mixture, season to taste and toss
5. Serve garnished with the basil or sage leaves

PENNE WITH BROCCOLI
Preparation time: 5–10 minutes
Cooking time: 10–15 minutes

400–500g broccoli
400g penne
4 tbsp olive oil
1 medium onion, finely sliced
4–5 garlic cloves, finely sliced
1 green chilli, sliced
fresh flat-leaf parsley
freshly ground black pepper

1. Cut the stalk off the broccoli, peel and cut it into thin slices, and cut the head into small florets
2. Cook the pasta in plenty of boiling water according to the instructions on the packet, then drain and keep warm if necessary
3. Heat the olive oil in a frying pan and sauté the onion for 2–3 minutes, then add the garlic and chilli and continue to sauté for another minute
4. Add the broccoli, stir to coat in the oil and sauté, stirring occasionally for about 6–7 minutes until the broccoli is cooked through but still firm, then stir through the chopped parsley,

season with black pepper and add a little extra olive oil if necessary

5. Divide the pasta among four serving plates and top with the broccoli

Variation: stir through 1–2 tbsp olive tapenade (see page 233) just before serving

PENNE WITH PEAS AND ARTICHOKES
Preparation time: 5 minutes
Cooking time: 15 minutes

400g penne
1 cup fresh or frozen peas
3 tbsp olive oil
2–3 garlic cloves
6–8 spring onions, chopped
1 cup mint leaves, chopped
150g bottled artichoke hearts, drained and halved
freshly ground black pepper

1. Bring a pan of water to a rolling boil, add the penne and cook according to the instructions on the packet
2. While the pasta is cooking, if using fresh peas, cook them in boiling water for 2–3 minutes, then drain
3. Heat the olive oil in a frying pan, add the garlic, spring onions and mint leaves and sauté for about 2 minutes, then add the peas and artichokes and cook until they are heated through
4. Put the pasta into a serving bowl, top with the sauce, season with black pepper and toss

PENNE WITH ZUCCHINI AND TOMATO
Preparation time: 5–10 minutes
Cooking time: 10 minutes

3–4 tbsp olive oil
1 onion, chopped
4 garlic cloves, chopped
1 green chilli, sliced
4–5 medium zucchini, sliced into fine 'matchsticks'
2 large tomatoes, chopped

1 cup fresh flat-leaf parsley or coriander, chopped
freshly ground black pepper
400g dried penne

1. Heat 3 tablespoons of the olive oil in a frying pan and sauté the onion for 2–3 minutes until translucent
2. Add the garlic and chilli and sauté briefly, then add the zucchini, stir to coat in the oil and continue to sauté for 1–2 minutes
3. Add the chopped tomato, stir to mix well and cook for another 3–4 minutes, then stir through the chopped parsley or coriander and additional olive oil if necessary and season with black pepper
4. Meanwhile, cook the pasta in plenty of boiling water according to the instructions on the packet, drain and serve topped with the zucchini sauce

RICE NOODLES WITH CURRIED PRAWNS
Preparation time: 10 minutes
Cooking time: 8–10 minutes

200g rice vermicelli noodles
2 tbsp olive oil
1 tbsp ground cumin
1 tbsp ground coriander
1 tsp turmeric
1 tsp cayenne pepper
2–3 garlic cloves, crushed
1 red chilli
1 red pepper, sliced
1 cup broccoli florets
16–20 raw tiger prawns
8 spring onions
1 tbsp lime juice
3 tbsp light soya sauce
fresh coriander

1. Put the noodles in a bowl, cover with boiling water and leave to stand for 5–6 minutes or cook according to the instructions on the packet, then drain and keep warm if necessary

2. While the noodles are soaking, heat the olive oil and fry the spices, garlic and chilli for 1 minute, then add the red pepper and broccoli and stir-fry for 2–3 minutes
3. Add the prawns and continue to fry until the prawns have just turned pink (about 2–3 minutes), then add the spring onions, lime juice and soya sauce and continue to cook for another minute (do not overcook the prawns or they will go tough)
4. Divide the noodles among four plates, top with the prawns and vegetables and garnish with fresh coriander

RICE NOODLES WITH PRAWNS AND MANGETOUT
Preparation time: 10 minutes
Cooking time: 8 minutes

150g rice vermicelli noodles
2 tbsp olive oil
2–3 garlic cloves, sliced
2 tsp chilli sambal
250g peeled raw prawns
400g mangetout, sliced
3–4 spring onions, sliced
2 tbsp lemon juice
1 tbsp fish sauce
½ cup fresh mint, chopped
½ cup fresh coriander, chopped

1. Put the noodles in a bowl, cover with boiling water and leave to stand for 5–6 minutes or according to the instructions on the packet
2. Heat the olive oil and sauté the garlic and chilli sambal for 1 minute
3. Add the prawns and stir-fry for 3–4 minutes until they become pink
4. Add the mangetout, spring onions, lemon juice and fish sauce and continue to stir-fry for another 1–2 minutes, then stir through the mint and coriander
5. Divide the noodles among the plates and top with the prawns and mangetout

SINGAPORE NOODLES

Preparation time: 10 minutes plus 30 minutes to marinate
Cooking time: 10 minutes

2–3 garlic cloves, crushed
1 tbsp grated fresh ginger
¼ cup oyster sauce
¼ cup soya sauce
2 chicken breasts, skinned and thinly sliced
400g dried rice vermicelli
2 tbsp vegetable oil
1 ½ tsp curry powder
2 celery stalks, julienned
1 large carrot, julienned
4 spring onions, thickly sliced
1 cup bean sprouts
½ cup fresh coriander, chopped
½ tsp sesame oil

1. Combine the garlic, ginger, 1 tablespoon oyster sauce and 2 teaspoons soya sauce in a nonmetallic bowl, add the chicken, toss to coat it in the marinade and leave for at least 30 minutes
2. Soak the noodles in boiling water for 5–6 minutes or until they are soft, then drain
3. Heat a wok, add the oil and stir-fry the curry powder, then add the chicken, with the marinade, and continue to stir-fry for 2–3 minutes until it has all changed colour and is just cooked through
4. Add the celery, carrot and spring onion and fry for another minute, then add the noodles and stir through
5. Add the bean sprouts, fresh coriander and sesame oil and remaining oyster sauce and soya sauce, and heat through for 1 minute

SPAGHETTI WITH MUSHROOMS

Preparation time: 10–15 minutes
Cooking time: 10 minutes

400g spaghetti
3 tbsp olive oil

2–3 garlic cloves, chopped
1 small red chilli, finely sliced
400–500g mixed mushrooms, peeled and sliced
pinch of salt
1 cup fresh flat-leaf parsley, chopped
1 tbsp lemon juice
freshly ground black pepper

1. Cook the spaghetti in plenty of boiling water according to the instructions on the packet, then drain
2. Heat the olive oil and briefly fry the garlic and chilli, then add the mushrooms and a pinch of salt and stir-fry briskly for about 4–5 minutes
3. Stir through the parsley and lemon juice and season with black pepper; add a little extra olive oil if necessary
4. Divide the pasta among four dishes and top with the mushrooms

SPAGHETTI WITH ROCKET AND CHERRY TOMATOES
Preparation time: 5 minutes
Cooking time: 5–10 minutes

400g dry spaghetti
4 tbsp olive oil
4 garlic cloves, sliced
1 large red chilli
250g cherry tomatoes, halved
10–12 spring onions, sliced
6 sun-blush tomatoes, chopped
2 cups rocket leaves
1 cup basil leaves, torn

1. Cook the pasta in plenty of boiling water according to the instructions on the packet
2. Heat 2 tablespoons of the olive oil in a frying pan and sauté the garlic and chilli for 1 minute, then add the cherry tomatoes and continue to sauté for another minute
3. Add the spring onions and sun-blush tomatoes, stir through and sauté for another 2–3 minutes
4. Take the pan off the heat, stir through the rocket and basil and pour over the extra olive oil

5. Divide the pasta among the serving bowls and top with the tomato sauce

SPAGHETTI WITH SPINACH AND WALNUTS
Preparation time: 15 minutes
Cooking time: 15 minutes

400g spaghetti
1 cup roughly chopped walnuts
2 tbsp olive oil
3–4 garlic cloves, sliced
8–10 spring onions, coarsely sliced
350g baby spinach leaves
zest of 1 lemon
½ cup flat-leaf parsley or coriander
freshly ground black pepper

1. Bring a large saucepan of water to a rolling boil, add the spaghetti and cook according to the instructions on the packet, then drain
2. Meanwhile, dry-fry the walnuts for 3–4 minutes, stirring frequently, then remove them from the pan
3. Heat the olive oil in a frying pan, add the garlic and spring onions and sauté for 1–2 minutes, then add the spinach, cover and cook until just wilted (about 1 minute)
4. Stir in the lemon zest, parsley or coriander and season with black pepper
5. Put the spaghetti in a serving dish, add the spinach and walnuts and toss

SPAGHETTI WITH ZUCCHINI AND PEAS
Preparation time: 5 minutes
Cooking time: 10 minutes

400g spaghetti or linguine
3 tbsp olive oil
4 garlic cloves, crushed
1 green chilli, chopped (optional)
4 medium zucchini, scrubbed and thinly sliced
2 cups frozen or fresh peas

½ cup white wine or chicken stock
2 tbsp lemon juice
4–5 spring onions, sliced
½ cup basil leaves
freshly ground black pepper

1. Cook the spaghetti in plenty of boiling water following the instructions on the packet, and drain
2. Heat the olive oil and sauté the garlic and chilli for about 10 seconds
3. Add the zucchini and continue to sauté for 1–2 minutes then add the peas and continue to cook for another minute
4. Add the wine or stock and lemon juice and simmer for about 5 minutes until the zucchini is soft
5. Add the spring onions and basil, stir and simmer for 1 minute
6. Add the zucchini and peas to the pasta, toss to mix well and season with black pepper; add a little extra olive oil if necessary

VEGETARIAN PAD THAI
Preparation time: 20 minutes
Cooking time: 10–15 minutes

400g dried rice noodles
¼ cup soya sauce
1 tbsp fish sauce
2 tbsp fresh lime juice
2 tsp chilli sambal
1 tbsp peanut oil
1 red onion, finely sliced
3–4 garlic cloves, sliced
1 small red pepper, sliced
12 mangetout, sliced
6 spring onions, sliced
1 cup bean sprouts
½ cup fresh coriander, chopped
¼ cup roasted unsalted peanuts, crushed (optional)

1. Soak the noodles in boiling water according to the instructions on the packet, then drain and set aside
2. Combine the soya sauce, fish sauce, lime juice and chilli sambal

3. Heat the oil in a wok, add the onion and stir-fry for 2–3 minutes, then add the garlic, red pepper and mangetout and continue to sauté for another 1–2 minutes
4. Add the noodles to the pan, stir through the spring onions, bean sprouts and coriander, pour over the sauce and toss to coat the noodles, then stir-fry for 1–2 minutes to heat through
5. Serve immediately and sprinkle with roasted peanuts

RICE

Rice is the basis for many delicious meals in the Mediterranean, Middle East and Asia. Rice is served with almost every meal throughout Asia, including breakfast.

ASPARAGUS AND BROAD BEAN RISOTTO
Preparation time: 10–15 minutes
Cooking time: 20 minutes

1–1 ½ litres chicken stock
2 tbsp olive oil
1 onion, finely chopped
3–4 garlic cloves, crushed
2 cups Arborio rice
1 cup white wine
1 cup podded fresh or frozen broad beans, peeled
8–12 asparagus spears, cut into four
8 marinated artichoke hearts, drained and cut in half
½ cup fresh mint leaves, chopped
freshly ground black pepper

1. Heat the stock to a gentle simmer
2. Sauté the onion in the olive oil for 3–4 minutes, then add the garlic and rice and continue to sauté for another minute
3. Add the wine and stir until the liquid is absorbed, then slowly add the chicken stock, a cup at a time, stirring continuously until the rice is cooked (you may need to slightly adjust the quantity of stock to ensure the rice is cooked through but not too moist)
4. Add the beans, asparagus and artichokes with the last cup of

stock and continue to cook until the rice and vegetables are all cooked

5. Stir through the mint and season with black pepper

BAKED PUMPKIN RISOTTO
Preparation time: 10 minutes
Cooking time: 30–40 minutes

1 ½ cups Arborio rice
3 cups chicken stock
3 tbsp olive oil
500g pumpkin, peeled, seeded and finely diced
2 tbsp flat-leaf parsley, chopped
freshly ground black pepper

1. Preheat the oven to 190°C
2. Put the rice, stock, olive oil and pumpkin into an oven-proof dish, cover tightly and bake in the oven for about 30 minutes or until the rice is soft, stirring occasionally (if necessary add a little more stock or water if the rice is not quite cooked)
3. Remove from the oven, stir through the parsley and season with black pepper

LEEK, PEA AND ASPARAGUS RISOTTO
Preparation time: 5 minutes
Cooking time: 30 minutes

2 ½ cups chicken stock
2 tbsp olive oil
½ onion, sliced
2 leeks, washed and finely sliced
4 garlic cloves, crushed
½ tsp turmeric (or saffron)
1 cup risotto rice
8 asparagus stalks, sliced into 1cm lengths
1 cup fresh or frozen peas
freshly ground black pepper
1 tbsp lemon juice
½ cup fresh basil leaves, shredded

1. Heat the stock to a gentle simmer
2. In a separate pan, sauté the onion and leek in the olive oil for 3–4 minutes until they are transparent, then add the garlic and turmeric and continue to sauté for another minute
3. Add the rice and stir to coat the rice in the oil, then slowly add the chicken stock, one cup at a time, stirring until the rice is soft but still has a bite to it (this may not require all the stock)
4. Add the peas and asparagus with the last cup of stock and continue to cook until the vegetables and rice are cooked
5. Season with black pepper and stir through the lemon juice and basil

Tip: Leftover risotto can be made into tasty risotto cakes. Shape the mixture into little balls, then shallow fry in olive oil until crispy golden and warmed through.

LEMON PILAU
This is a simple lemony-flavoured rice that is lovely served with grilled or poached fish.

Preparation time: 5 minutes
Cooking time: 12–13 minutes

1 ½ cups long-grain rice
2 ½ cups chicken or vegetable stock, or water
1 tbsp lemon rind
3 tbsp fresh lemon juice
½ cup mixed chopped fresh herbs (coriander, basil, mint, thyme, oregano)
freshly ground black pepper

1. Rinse the rice under running water, let it drain, then put it in a saucepan with the stock, lemon rind and lemon juice; bring to the boil, then reduce the heat, cover the pan and cook gently for 12 minutes or until all the liquid has been absorbed and the rice is cooked through (if the rice is not quite cooked add a little extra water and continue cooking)
2. Stir through the herbs and season with black pepper

RABBIT PILAF
Preparation time: 10 minutes
Cooking time: 40–45 minutes

½ tsp ground coriander
½ tsp ground cumin
¼ tsp turmeric
½ tsp cayenne pepper
1 tsp paprika
¼ tsp ground cinnamon
½ tsp coarse black pepper
1 tbsp lemon juice
3 tbsp olive oil
2 rabbit portions, skinned, boned and cut into 2cm pieces
1 onion, finely chopped
3–4 garlic cloves, sliced
4 medium vine-ripened tomatoes, chopped
½ cup raisins
¼ cup dried apricots, chopped
1 cup short-grain rice
2 cups chicken stock
½ cup mint, chopped
½ cup coriander, chopped
1 tbsp pine nuts
1 tbsp flaked almonds

1. Mix together all the dry spices with the lemon juice and 1 tablespoon of the olive oil in a bowl, add the rabbit pieces and stir to coat in the spices, then leave to marinate for at least 30 minutes
2. Heat the remaining oil, add the rabbit and marinade and sauté until it has changed colour, then remove from the pan and keep warm
3. Add the onion to the pan and sauté for 3–4 minutes, add the garlic and continue to sauté for another minute, then add the rabbit, chopped tomatoes, raisins, apricots and rice, stir to coat everything in the oil, pour over the chicken stock, bring to the boil, cover and simmer for about 25 minutes; remove from the heat and leave to stand for about 5 minutes

4. Stir through the coriander and mint and sprinkle with pine nuts and almonds

Variation: use chicken, prawns or lamb

SEAFOOD PAELLA
Preparation time: 15–20 minutes
Cooking time: 30 minutes

2–3 tbsp olive oil
1 medium red onion, sliced
4–5 garlic cloves, finely chopped
1 red chilli, sliced (or to taste)
1 tsp turmeric
1 tsp cayenne pepper
1 cup paella rice, washed and drained
2 cups chicken or vegetable stock
1 red pepper, seeded and sliced
12–16 cherry tomatoes, halved
4 large unshelled green prawns (optional)
500g fresh mussels
100g shelled raw prawns
6 small squid, cut into rings
100g small scallops
16 mangetout, cut in half
4–5 marinated artichoke hearts, each cut into about 3 pieces
2 large handfuls (90g) baby spinach leaves
1 cup fresh flat-leaf parsley or coriander, chopped
freshly ground black pepper

1. Heat the olive oil and sauté the onion for 2–3 minutes, then add the garlic, chilli, turmeric and cayenne pepper and sauté for another minute
2. Add the rice, stir to coat with the oil and continue to sauté for another minute
3. Add the stock, cover and simmer gently for about 15 minutes until the rice is soft
4. Add the red pepper, tomatoes and large prawns, stir through the rice, cover the pan and simmer for another 5 minutes
5. Add the mussels and prawns and continue to simmer for another 2–3 minutes, then add the scallops, squid, mangetout,

artichoke hearts and spinach, stir to mix well and sauté for another 2–3 minutes until all the seafood is just cooked through and the spinach has wilted

6. Stir through the parsley or coriander and season with black pepper

SPICY BASMATI RICE

This spicy rice is good with plain grilled chicken or vegetables.

Preparation time: 5 minutes
Cooking time: 15 minutes

1 ½ cups basmati rice
1 tbsp olive oil
2 tsp ground coriander
1 tsp ground cumin
1 tsp cayenne pepper
2 garlic cloves, chopped
2 ½ cups chicken or vegetable stock, or water
½ cup fresh coriander leaves
freshly ground black pepper

1. Rinse the rice under running water
2. Heat the olive oil in a saucepan; add the spices and garlic and sauté for about 1 minute until the spices are fragrant
3. Add the rice and stir to coat in the oil, then add the stock and bring to a boil; reduce the heat to a minimum, cover and cook for 12 minutes or until all the liquid has been absorbed (if the rice is not quite cooked add a little extra water and continue cooking)
4. Remove from the heat, stir through the coriander and season with black pepper

ZUCCHINI AND PEA RISOTTO

Preparation time: 10 minutes
Cooking time: 20–30 minutes

1 litre chicken or vegetable stock
2 tbsp olive oil
1 medium onion, chopped
4 garlic cloves, chopped

1 green chilli, sliced
2 medium zucchini, finely chopped
2 cups fresh or frozen peas
1 cup Arborio rice
¼ cup dry vermouth or dry white wine (optional)
zest from one small lemon
2 tbsp lemon juice
2 cups baby spinach leaves
2 tbsp chopped fresh mint leaves
2 tbsp chopped fresh flat-leaf parsley

1. Heat the stock to a gentle simmer
2. In a separate saucepan heat the olive oil and sauté the onion for 2–3 minutes, add the garlic, chilli, zucchini and fresh peas, stir to coat in the oil and continue to sauté for another 2–3 minutes until the zucchini has softened, then add the rice and stir to coat in the oil
3. Add the vermouth or wine and a little of the stock, stirring until the liquid is absorbed, then gradually add the rest of the stock, one cupful at a time, until the rice is soft but still has a bite to it (this may not require all the stock – stir frequently to stop the rice sticking to the bottom of the pan)
4. Add the lemon zest, lemon juice, spinach and chopped mint (add frozen peas at this stage), stir through and cook for another 1–2 minutes until the peas are cooked and the spinach wilted, then stir through the chopped parsley

MEAN BEANS

BEAN CURD AND TOFU

OTHER LEGUMES

Beans include:

- *soya beans, including bean curd, tofu, tempeh etc.*
- *other legumes, including peas, cannellini beans, lentils, chick-peas, red kidney beans, bollotti beans etc.*

BEAN CURD AND TOFU

Bean curd, tofu and tempeh have an unusual texture and some people find them tasteless, but they absorb flavours well and quickly, require no lengthy cooking and are very easily digested.

BEAN CURD WITH CHILLI AND SPRING ONIONS
Preparation time: 5 minutes
Cooking time: 5 minutes

500g soft bean curd
4 spring onions, thinly sliced
1 red chilli, thinly sliced
2 tbsp chopped fresh coriander
2 tbsp light soya sauce
3 tbsp olive oil
1 tbsp sesame oil

1. Cut the bean curd into cubes and place in a serving dish
2. Scatter the spring onion, chilli and coriander over the bean curd and pour over the soya sauce
3. Warm the oils then pour them over the bean curd

Serve with steamed rice

STIR-FRIED TOFU WITH BOK CHOY
Preparation time: 5 minutes plus 10 minutes to marinate
Cooking time: 5–10 minutes

500g firm tofu, drained and diced
1 tbsp grated fresh ginger
2 tbsp soya sauce
500g baby bok choy, sliced
2 tbsp vegetable oil
1 red onion, thinly sliced
4 garlic cloves, crushed

1 tbsp chilli sambal
1 tbsp sweet chilli sauce
1 tbsp sesame oil
1 tbsp toasted sesame seeds

1. Put the tofu and ginger in a bowl, pour over the soya sauce and leave for 10 minutes
2. Steam the bok choy for 2–3 minutes, then drain and keep warm
3. Heat a wok, add the vegetable oil and stir-fry the onion for 3–4 minutes, then add the garlic, chilli sambal and chilli sauce and continue to sauté for another minute
4. Add the tofu with the marinade and simmer for 2–3 minutes until heated through, then add the bok choy, soya sauce and sesame oil, stir gently to mix and heat for another minute
5. Serve sprinkled with the sesame seeds

STIR-FRIED TOFU WITH MANGETOUT AND CHINESE MUSHROOMS
Preparation time: 10–15 minutes
Cooking time: 15 minutes

4 tbsp vegetable oil
500g firm tofu, drained and cubed
2 tsp chilli sambal
3 garlic cloves, finely chopped
300g mangetout
400g fresh shiitake mushrooms, sliced
1 tbsp water
½ cup coriander
freshly ground black pepper

1. Heat 2 tablespoons of the oil in a wok and stir-fry the tofu for 2–3 minutes each side until lightly browned, then remove from the pan and keep warm
2. Heat the remaining oil in the wok, add the chilli, garlic, mangetout, mushrooms and water and stir-fry for 1–2 minutes until the vegetables are just cooked
3. Add the tofu to the pan and stir gently
4. Serve garnished with fresh coriander and season with black pepper

SWEET AND SOUR TOFU
Preparation time: 10–15 minutes
Cooking time: 20 minutes

1 tbsp sweet chilli sauce
2 tbsp tomato sauce
2 tbsp brown rice vinegar
2 tbsp light soya sauce
1 cup chicken or vegetable stock
3 tbsp vegetable oil
500g firm tofu, drained and cubed
4 garlic cloves, crushed
1 tbsp grated fresh ginger
1 red chilli, sliced
1 carrot, julienned
8–10 baby mushrooms, thickly sliced
2 stalks celery, thickly sliced
1 tbsp cornflour
100g mangetout halved
6–8 spring onions, thickly sliced
1 cup bean sprouts

1. Combine the sweet chilli sauce, tomato sauce, vinegar, soya sauce and stock in a small bowl
2. Heat 2 tablespoons of the vegetable oil in a wok and stir-fry the tofu for 2 minutes each side until crisp and golden, then drain on kitchen paper and keep warm
3. Wipe the wok clean, then add the remaining oil and add the garlic, ginger and chilli and stir-fry for 1 minute; add the carrot, mushrooms and celery and continue to stir-fry for another minute
4. Add the sauce (from step 1) and simmer gently for 2–3 minutes until the vegetables are soft
5. Mix the cornflour to a smooth paste with a little water, then add to the wok with the mangetout, spring onions and bean sprouts and cook until the sauce thickens
6. Divide the tofu among the serving bowls and spoon over the sauce

TOFU AND PUMPKIN RED CURRY

Preparation time: 15 minutes
Cooking time: 20 minutes

3 tbsp vegetable oil
350g firm tofu, drained
1 medium red onion, sliced
2 garlic cloves, crushed
1 tbsp grated fresh ginger
4 lime leaves
1–2 tbsp red curry paste (page 237)
400g pumpkin, peeled, seeded and chopped
1 cup coconut milk
½ cup vegetable or chicken stock
2 tbsp fish sauce
1 cup bean sprouts
½ cup bamboo shoots
1–2 tbsp lime juice
½ cup fresh coriander, chopped

1. Heat 1 tablespoon of the vegetable oil and fry the tofu for 1–2 minutes each side, then remove from the pan, cut into cubes and keep warm
2. Heat the remaining oil and stir-fry the onion for 3–4 minutes, then add the garlic, ginger, lime leaves and curry paste and continue to fry for another minute
3. Add the pumpkin and stir to coat in the paste; continue frying for 3 minutes, then add the coconut milk, stir through and simmer for another minute
4. Add the stock and fish sauce and continue to simmer until the pumpkin is cooked, then add the tofu, bean sprouts and bamboo shoots and heat through for another minute
5. Stir through the lime juice and garnish with fresh coriander

TOFU WITH ASIAN GREENS

Preparation time: 10–15 minutes
Cooking time: 15 minutes

4 tbsp olive oil
1 onion, thinly sliced

3 garlic cloves, crushed
1 tbsp grated fresh ginger
1 tsp cayenne pepper
500g baby bok choy, sliced lengthways
300g choi sum, cut into thirds
200g green beans, sliced
½ cup teriyaki sauce
500g firm tofu, drained and cubed
1 tbsp sesame oil
½ cup fresh coriander, chopped

1. Heat a wok, add two tablespoons of the olive oil and cook the onion for 2–3 minutes, then add the garlic, ginger and cayenne pepper and continue to fry for 30 seconds
2. Add the vegetables and stir-fry for 2–3 minutes, then add the teriyaki sauce, cover the pan and simmer for 2–3 minutes until the vegetables are cooked
3. Add the tofu and sesame oil and simmer for 2 minutes turning once (the tofu will break up) and serve garnished with fresh coriander

TOFU WITH CHINESE MUSHROOMS
Preparation time: 5 minutes
Cooking time: 10 minutes

500g soft tofu, cut into four pieces
2 tbsp olive oil
3–4 garlic cloves, crushed
1 tbsp ginger, grated
1 red chilli, sliced
3 celery stalks, sliced
6 spring onions, sliced
125g fresh shiitake mushrooms, sliced
1 cup chicken stock
1 tbsp mirin or Chinese cooking wine
4 tbsp light soya sauce
1 tbsp cornflour
½ cup fresh coriander, chopped

1. Steam the tofu until heated through or put the tofu into a deep dish, pour over boiling water and leave until it is heated through, then drain

2. Heat the olive oil and stir-fry the garlic, ginger and chilli for 1 minute, then add the celery, spring onions and mushrooms, chicken stock, mirin and soya sauce, bring to a gentle simmer, cover and simmer for 2–3 minutes until the vegetables are just tender

3. Mix the cornflour to a smooth paste with a little water, add to the stock and simmer gently for another minute

4. Divide the tofu among the plates and cover with the mushroom sauce

5. Serve garnished with coriander

OTHER LEGUMES

BAKED CANNELLINI BEANS WITH TOMATOES
Preparation time: 5 minutes
Cooking time: 30 minutes

1 × 400g tin cannellini beans, rinsed and drained
2 garlic cloves, sliced
1 tsp chilli sambal
1 small red onion, finely sliced
200g cherry tomatoes, halved
2 tbsp olive oil
fresh basil leaves, torn
freshly ground black pepper

1. Preheat the oven to 200°C
2. Put the beans, garlic, chilli, onion and tomatoes into a baking dish, pour over the olive oil and stir to coat all the vegetables and beans in the oil
3. Cover with foil and bake for 25–30 minutes or until the vegetables are cooked
4. Sprinkle with the fresh basil and season with black pepper

CHICKPEAS WITH AUBERGINE
Preparation time: 10 minutes
Cooking time: 15 minutes

3 tbsp olive oil
1 red onion, chopped

4–6 garlic cloves, crushed
1 red chilli, chopped, or 1 tsp cayenne pepper
2 tsp ground coriander
2 tsp ground cumin
1 tsp paprika
1 medium aubergine, cut into 1cm cubes
4–5 medium vine-ripened tomatoes, chopped
4 tbsp lemon juice
1 × 400g tin chickpeas, rinsed and drained
½ cup fresh coriander, chopped
2 tbsp fresh mint, chopped

1. Heat the oil and sauté the onion for 2–3 minutes, then add the garlic, chilli and dry spices and continue to sauté for another minute
2. Add the aubergine, tomatoes and lemon juice and simmer gently for 5–10 minutes
3. Add the chickpeas and simmer for another 5 minutes
4. Stir through the coriander and mint and leave to cool to room temperature

CURRIED CHICKPEAS WITH SPINACH AND TOMATO

Preparation time: 10 minutes
Cooking time: 10 minutes

2 tbsp olive oil
1 large red onion, finely chopped
3–4 garlic cloves, thinly sliced
1 tbsp grated fresh ginger
1 red chilli, finely sliced, or 2 tsp chilli sambal
2 tsp ground cumin
1 tsp turmeric
1 tsp ground black pepper
1 red pepper, seeded and diced
2 cups fresh or frozen sweet corn kernels
1 × 400g can chickpeas, rinsed and drained
2 tbsp water
200g cherry tomatoes, halved
100g baby spinach leaves
1 cup fresh coriander, chopped

1. Heat the olive oil in a wok or large sauté pan and sauté the onion for 2–3 minutes
2. Add the garlic, ginger, chilli, cumin, turmeric and black pepper and sauté for another minute
3. Add the red pepper and sweet corn, stir to coat in the oil, and continue to sauté for another minute, then add the chickpeas and water and continue to cook for another 3–4 minutes
4. Add the tomatoes and continue cooking for 2–3 minutes until they are soft
5. Stir through the spinach and continue to cook until the leaves have just wilted, then stir through the coriander and serve immediately

LENTILS WITH SPINACH
Preparation time: 5 minutes
Cooking time: 20–25 minutes

1 cup green or brown lentils, washed
4 tbsp olive oil
1 medium onion, chopped
1 tsp ground coriander
1 tsp cayenne pepper
180g baby spinach leaves
2 tbsp lemon juice
freshly ground black pepper

1. Put the lentils in a saucepan, cover with water and simmer for about 20 minutes until they are cooked (add a little more water if necessary)
2. Meanwhile heat 2 tablespoons of the olive oil in a sauté pan with a lid and sauté the onion for 3–4 minutes until soft, then add the ground coriander and cayenne pepper and cook for another minute
3. Add the spinach, sprinkle over the lemon juice, cover and cook for about a minute until it has just wilted
4. Stir the spinach and onion and remaining olive oil through the lentils and season with black pepper

RED LENTIL DHAL
Preparation time: 10 minutes
Cooking time: 25–30 minutes

2 tbsp vegetable oil
1 cinnamon stick
4–5 cloves
4–5 cardamom pods, crushed
1 onion, finely chopped
2 garlic cloves, crushed
1 tbsp grated fresh ginger
1 tsp garam masala
1 tsp cayenne pepper
1 cup red lentils
1 tbsp lemon juice

1. Heat the vegetable oil and briefly fry the cinnamon stick, cloves and cardamom pods, then add the onion and fry for 3–4 minutes
2. Add the garlic, ginger, garam masala and cayenne pepper and fry for another minute, then add the lentils and stir to coat in the oil
3. Add enough water to cover the lentils by about 2cm, bring to a boil, then reduce the heat and simmer for about 20 minutes until the lentils are cooked (add a little more water if necessary), then stir through the lemon juice

RED PEPPERS WITH KIDNEY BEANS
Preparation time: 10 minutes
Cooking time: 20 minutes

4 tbsp olive oil
1 large red onion, chopped
4 garlic cloves, crushed
1 tsp ground cumin
1 tsp ground coriander
1 tsp paprika
1 tbsp harissa or 2 tsp chilli sambal (or to taste)
2 red peppers, seeded, and coarsely chopped
400g tinned tomatoes, chopped

2 celery stalks, finely sliced
400g tinned red kidney beans, drained and rinsed
freshly ground black pepper
½ cup fresh coriander, chopped
½ cup fresh mint, chopped

1. Heat the olive oil in a large frying pan and sauté the onion for 3–4 minutes, then add the garlic, ground cumin, ground coriander, paprika and harissa and sauté for another minute
2. Add the red peppers, stir to coat in the oil and sauté for 3–4 minutes, then add the tomatoes, celery and red kidney beans, season with black pepper and simmer gently for about 15 minutes until everything is heated through
3. Stir through the coriander and mint and serve

SENSUOUS SEAFOOD

BAKED COD WITH SPINACH, FENNEL AND TOMATO
Preparation time: 10 minutes
Cooking time: 15–20 minutes

4 small pieces of cod
2–3 garlic cloves, sliced
3–4 vine-ripened tomatoes, sliced
½ large fennel bulb, sliced
120g baby spinach leaves
1 tsp fennel seeds, crushed
freshly ground black pepper
1 tbsp lemon juice
2 tbsp olive oil

1. Preheat the oven to 200°C
2. Place the fish, garlic, tomatoes, fennel and spinach in an oven-proof dish, sprinkle over the crushed fennel seeds and season with black pepper
3. Shake the lemon juice and olive oil together and pour over the fish
4. Cover and bake for 15–20 minutes until the fish is cooked through

BAKED FISH WITH SOYA SAUCE
Preparation time: 2–3 minutes plus 15 minutes marinating time
Cooking time: 5–6 minutes

2 tsp fresh lime juice
4 garlic cloves, crushed
1 small red chilli, chopped
2 tbsp mirin or Chinese cooking wine
3 tbsp light soya sauce
4 fillets cod or other firm-fleshed white fish
½ cup fresh coriander, chopped

1. Shake the lime juice, garlic, chilli, mirin and soya sauce together
2. Put the fish into a baking dish or frying pan, pour over the marinade and leave for about 15 minutes
3. Bake covered or poach the fish in the marinade for about 5–6 minutes or until the fish is just cooked
4. Serve garnished with coriander

CHILLI PRAWNS
Preparation time: 5 minutes
Cooking time: 8–10 minutes

2 tbsp olive oil
1 small onion, chopped
3–4 garlic cloves, crushed
1 tbsp grated fresh ginger
1–2 long red chillies, sliced
¼ cup tomato sauce
1 tbsp sweet chilli sauce or chilli sauce
2 tbsp mirin or Chinese cooking wine
1 tbsp light soya sauce
500g raw prawns
3 tbsp coriander, chopped
4 spring onions, sliced

1. Heat the olive oil in a wok and stir-fry the onion for 2–3 minutes, then add the garlic, ginger and chilli and continue to stir-fry for another minute
2. Add the tomato sauce, chilli sauce, mirin and soya sauce, and continue to stir-fry for another minute (if the sauce is too thick add a little water)
3. Add the prawns, stir to ensure they are well coated in the sauce and continue to stir-fry until the prawns turn pink, then stir through the coriander and spring onions

FISH CURRY
Preparation time: 10 minutes
Cooking time: 10–12 minutes

2 tbsp olive oil
1 large onion, sliced
3–4 garlic cloves, crushed
1 tbsp grated fresh ginger
1 tsp turmeric
1 stalk lemon grass, cut into 3–4 pieces and slightly crushed
3–4 lime leaves
1 green chilli
2 tbsp Thai fish sauce

2 tbsp brown rice vinegar
1 cup coconut milk
¼ cup water
2 vine-ripened tomatoes, chopped
1 cup green beans, sliced
8–10 baby mushrooms, halved
4 pieces swordfish or other firm white fish
1 cup fresh coriander, chopped

1. Heat the olive oil and fry the onion for 2–3 minutes, then add the garlic, ginger, turmeric, lemon grass, lime leaves and chilli and fry for another minute
2. Add the fish sauce, vinegar, coconut milk and water, and simmer for 2–3 minutes, then add all the vegetables and continue to simmer for 4–5 minutes until they are just tender
3. While the vegetables are cooking, poach or steam the fish for 4–5 minutes until it is just cooked, then drain and cut into cubes
4. Add the fish and coriander to the vegetables and stir gently to mix

FISH STEW
Preparation time: 10–15 minutes
Cooking time: 30 minutes

400g firm white fish (such as swordfish)
5–6 baby squid tubes
250g raw tiger prawns, peeled
500g fresh mussels
2 tbsp olive oil
2 small red onions, finely sliced
4–5 garlic cloves, chopped
2 red chillies, chopped
1 stalk lemon grass, cut into 3–4 pieces and slightly crushed
3–4 lime leaves
½ tsp ground cumin
1 tsp paprika
1 tbsp tomato paste
3 medium to large vine-ripened tomatoes, chopped
2–3 medium white potatoes, diced
600ml chicken or vegetable stock

8–12 button mushrooms
1 cup mangetout, halved
fresh coriander

1. Prepare the fish and seafood: wash the swordfish and cut into largish chunks; wash the squid and cut into rings and halve the tentacles; clean the mussels and peel the prawns if necessary (although we always leave the tails on)
2. Heat the olive oil in a large pan and sauté the onion for 2–3 minutes, then add the garlic, chilli, lemon grass, lime leaves, ground cumin, paprika and tomato paste and continue to sauté for another minute
3. Add the tomatoes and potatoes, fry for another minute, then add the stock and simmer for about 15–20 minutes until the potatoes are soft
4. Add the mushrooms and mangetout, and simmer for another 2–3 minutes, then add the mussels, cover the pan and continue to cook for about 2 minutes, then add the fish and prawns, and continue cooking for another 2 minutes until the prawns have just turned pink and the mussels have opened
5. Add the squid, continue to cook for 1 minute, then stir through the coriander and serve immediately (it is important not to overcook the seafood or it will be tough and rubbery)

FRESH TUNA WITH NORI
Preparation time: 6–7 minutes
Cooking time: 4–5 minutes

4 tuna steaks (about 400g)
½ tsp wasabi paste
2–4 sheets of nori seaweed
light soya sauce

1. Spread a very thin layer of the wasabi paste on one side of the tuna
2. Wrap the tuna steaks tightly in a single layer of nori, trimming off any excess
3. Cook the tuna on a high heat in a griddle pan for 1–2 minutes each side (tuna becomes very tough if it is overcooked and it is best just lightly seared)
4. Slice the tuna into thin strips and sprinkle with light soya sauce

MUSSELS WITH LEMON GRASS
Preparation time: 15 minutes
Cooking time: 20–25 minutes

1 cup chicken stock
⅓ cup white wine
3–4 garlic cloves, finely chopped
1 tbsp grated fresh ginger
1 stalk lemon grass, cut into 3 or 4 pieces and slightly crushed
4–5 lime leaves
1–2 red chillies, sliced
4–6 spring onions, sliced
1 cup coconut milk
500g fresh mussels, cleaned
1 cup fresh coriander, chopped
2 tbsp lemon juice

1. Heat the stock and wine with the garlic, ginger, lemon grass, lime leaves, chilli and spring onions and simmer for about 15 minutes, then remove the lemon grass and lime leaves
2. Add the coconut milk and bring to a gentle simmer (do not boil) then add the cleaned mussels, cover and simmer for about 6–7 minutes until the mussels are just cooked (do not overcook or the mussels will be tough)
3. Stir through the lemon juice and coriander and serve in soup bowls

PLAICE WITH MUSHROOMS
Preparation time: 5 minutes
Cooking time: 5 minutes

2 tbsp olive oil
2 garlic cloves, sliced
½ tbsp grated fresh ginger
200g baby mushrooms, sliced
4 spring onions, thickly sliced
4 plaice fillets
½ cup chicken stock
1 tbsp light soya sauce
2 tbsp Chinese cooking wine

1 tsp sesame oil
fresh coriander

1. Heat the olive oil and sauté the garlic, ginger, mushrooms and spring onions for 1 minute
2. Add the plaice and continue to sauté for another 2–3 minutes until just cooked
3. Add the stock, soya sauce and rice wine and cook for another 1–2 minutes to heat through
4. Serve sprinkled with the sesame oil and fresh coriander

SALMON AND SWEET POTATO CAKES

We recommend salmon with bones as it is good for your calcium intake.

Preparation time: 15 minutes
Cooking time: 20 minutes

200g tinned red salmon with bones
½ cup self-raising flour
½ cup rice flour
¼ tsp turmeric
1–2 cups coconut milk
250g sweet potato, peeled and grated
1 red chilli, finely sliced
¼ cup flat-leaf parsley, finely chopped
2–3 tbsp chives, finely chopped
sunflower or groundnut oil for frying

1. Drain the salmon, remove any large pieces of skin and mash with a fork
2. Mix together the self-raising and rice flours and turmeric and gradually add the coconut milk to make a thick batter
3. Stir in the sweet potato, salmon, chilli, parsley and chives, and mix well (add more coconut milk if necessary, but be careful not to make the batter too thin)
4. Heat the oil in a wok and fry spoonfuls of the salmon and potato mix for 3–4 minutes each side until they are well browned on the outside and cooked through but soft inside
5. Drain on kitchen paper

These are delicious served with sweet chilli sauce.

SPICY TOMATO FISH
Preparation time: 5 minutes
Cooking time: 20 minutes

2 tbsp olive oil
2 small red onions, sliced
4 cloves of garlic, sliced
4 vine-ripened tomatoes, chopped
2 tbsp Thai fish sauce
2 tbsp brown rice vinegar
2 tbsp sweet chilli sauce
1 cup fresh coriander leaves, chopped
freshly ground black pepper
4 small pieces cod

1. Heat the olive oil and sauté the onion for 2–3 minutes, then add the garlic and continue to sauté for another minute
2. Add the tomatoes, fish sauce, rice vinegar and sweet chilli sauce and sauté for about 10–15 minutes; stir occasionally and press down on the tomato to break it up (add a little bit of water if the sauce becomes too thick)
3. Just before serving, stir through the coriander and season with black pepper
4. Meanwhile, in a separate pan poach or steam the fish for 5–6 minutes or until it is just cooked
5. Serve the fish on individual plates and top with the sauce

SQUID IN SOYA SAUCE
Preparation time: 5 minutes
Cooking time: 5 minutes

2 tbsp olive oil
3–4 garlic cloves, crushed
1 tbsp fresh ginger, grated
½ long red chilli, or to taste
500g baby squid, washed and cut into rings
1 tbsp light soya sauce

1. Heat the olive oil and stir-fry the garlic, ginger and chilli for 1 minute
2. Add the squid and continue to stir-fry for 1–2 minutes

3. Add the soya sauce and continue to cook for another minute (do not overcook or the squid will be tough)

STIR-FRIED PRAWNS WITH BEAN SPROUTS AND RED PEPPER
Preparation time: 20–30 minutes
Cooking time: 12–15 minutes

3 tbsp olive oil
1 red onion, sliced
3–4 garlic cloves, peeled and thinly sliced
2 tbsp grated fresh ginger
½ long red chilli, finely sliced
1 red pepper, seeded and sliced
300g peeled raw tiger prawns (5–6 prawns per person)
1 tbsp sesame oil
3 tbsp Chinese cooking wine or mirin
3 tbsp light soya sauce
350g fresh bean sprouts
½ cup fresh basil, torn
cup fresh coriander, chopped
4–6 spring onions, coarsely sliced

1. Heat the olive oil in a frying pan or wok, add the onion and stir-fry for 2–3 minutes
2. Add the garlic, ginger and chilli and continue to stir-fry for a minute, then add the red pepper and continue to stir-fry for another 1–2 minutes
3. Add the prawns and cook for about 3 minutes, stirring occasionally until the prawns have all just turned pink
4. Add the sesame oil, mirin or rice wine, soya sauce and bean sprouts, and toss and stir-fry for another 1–2 minutes
5. Finally, stir through the basil, coriander and spring onions

STIR-FRIED SCALLOPS WITH BOK CHOY AND MANGETOUT
Preparation time: 5 minutes plus 20 minutes to marinate
Cooking time: 5 minutes

2 tbsp rice wine
1 tbsp fresh ginger, grated
1 tbsp sesame oil

350g scallops
1 tbsp olive oil
2–3 garlic cloves, crushed
1 tsp sweet chilli sauce
200g bok choy
60g mangetout
4–6 spring onions, sliced
⅓ cup chicken stock
freshly ground black pepper
fresh coriander, chopped

1. Mix together 1 tablespoon rice wine, 1 teaspoon ginger and 1 teaspoon sesame oil, pour over the scallops and marinate for 15–20 minutes
2. Heat the remaining sesame oil and olive oil, and stir-fry the garlic and remaining ginger for 30 seconds, then add the chilli sauce, remaining rice wine, bok choy, mangetout and spring onions and cook for 2–3 minutes
3. Add the scallops, with the marinade and the chicken stock, cover and cook for 1–2 minutes until the scallops are just cooked
4. Season with black pepper and garnish with fresh coriander

STIR-FRIED SQUID IN BLACK BEAN SAUCE
Preparation time: 10 minutes
Cooking time: 8–10 minutes

8 small squid tubes
2 tbsp olive oil
1 small onion, finely sliced
2–3 garlic cloves, sliced
½ tbsp grated fresh ginger
1 tsp chilli sambal
1 small red pepper, seeded and cut into cubes
1 tsp black bean sauce
1 tbsp Chinese rice wine or mirin
1 tbsp sesame oil
2 tbsp chopped fresh coriander

1. Open up the squid tubes, score the inside with a crisscross pattern and cut into 2–3 pieces

2. Heat the olive oil and stir-fry the onion for 2–3 minutes, then add the garlic, ginger and chilli and continue to fry for another minute
3. Add the red pepper and black bean sauce and continue to stir-fry for another minute
4. Add the squid and rice wine and stir-fry for 1–2 minutes (don't overcook the squid or it will be tough and rubbery), then stir through the sesame oil and coriander

SWEET AND SOUR PRAWNS
Preparation time: 5 minutes plus 15 minutes to marinate
Cooking time: 6–8 minutes

1 tbsp sesame oil
1 tbsp grated fresh ginger
1 tbsp Chinese rice wine or mirin
250g raw tiger prawns, peeled
2 tbsp olive oil
2–3 garlic cloves sliced
2 tsp sweet chilli sauce
1 red pepper, seeded and diced
1 green pepper, seeded and diced
1 stalk celery, sliced
4–6 spring onions, sliced
2 tbsp tomato ketchup
1 tbsp brown rice vinegar
1 tsp light soya sauce
fresh coriander
freshly ground black pepper

1. Mix together the sesame oil, 1 teaspoon ginger and the rice wine, pour over the prawns and leave to marinate for about 15 minutes
2. Heat the olive oil and stir-fry the garlic, remaining ginger, chilli sauce and red and green peppers for 2–3 minutes until the pepper has softened
3. Add the prawns with the marinade and continue to stir-fry for 2–3 minutes until the prawns turn pink, then add the celery, spring onions, tomato ketchup, rice vinegar and soya sauce, and heat through
4. Garnish with fresh coriander and season with black pepper

SWORDFISH KEBABS
Preparation time: 5–10 minutes plus 20 minutes marinating time
Cooking time: 5 minutes

400–500g swordfish fillet, cut into cubes
1 red pepper, seeded and diced
Fresh bay or sage leaves
2–3 garlic cloves
1 red chilli, sliced
1 tbsp lemon juice
3 tbsp olive oil

1. Thread alternating pieces of swordfish and red pepper onto skewers, with an occasional bay or sage leaf
2. Process together the garlic, chilli, lemon juice and olive oil, pour over the fish and leave to marinate for about 20 minutes
3. Grill, turning from side to side for about 4–5 minutes until the fish is just cooked
4. Serve with salsa verde (page 236)

THAI-STYLE CURRIED COD WITH ORANGE PEPPERS
Preparation time: 20–30 minutes
Cooking time: 15–20 minutes

2 orange peppers, deseeded and sliced
1 large onion, coarsely chopped
7–8 garlic cloves, peeled
2½cm piece of ginger
2–3 red chillies
1 tbsp tamarind paste
4 pieces of cod or other firm white fish
2 tbsp olive oil
4 stalks lemon grass, cut into 5cm pieces and slightly crushed
6 lime leaves
2 tbsp turmeric
400ml coconut milk
½ cup chicken stock
60g green beans
1 cup frozen peas
100g baby spinach

60g mangetout
1 cup bean sprouts
¼ cup fresh coriander, chopped

1. Blend together the peppers, onion, garlic, ginger and chillies to a smooth paste in a food processor
2. Pour 2 tablespoons boiling water over the tamarind paste and leave it to soak, then strain, reserving the liquid
3. Heat the olive oil, add the pepper paste, lemon grass, lime leaves and turmeric and stir-fry for 2–3 minutes
4. Add the coconut milk and continue to stir-fry for another 2–3 minutes (at this point you can strain the liquid if you would prefer a smooth sauce)
5. Add the stock and green beans and simmer for 3–4 minutes
6. Add the peas and continue to simmer for another 1–2 minutes, then add the spinach, mangetout, bean sprouts and tamarind water and cook for another minute or until the spinach is just wilted
7. While the vegetables are cooking, poach or steam the cod in a separate pan for about 5–6 minutes or until cooked through, drain and keep warm if necessary
8. Place a piece of cod in each bowl, spoon over the vegetable sauce and garnish with coriander

POULTRY WITH PANACHE

CHICKEN

DUCK

CHICKEN

BAKED CHICKEN WITH FENNEL
Preparation time: 10 minutes
Cooking time: 30–35 minutes

4 chicken breasts, skinned
8 garlic cloves, peeled
2 fennel bulbs, sliced
1 tsp crushed fennel seeds
1 tsp coarse black pepper
2 tbsp lemon juice
2 tbsp olive oil
½ cup chicken stock or white wine

1. Preheat the oven to 190°C
2. Place the chicken, garlic and fennel in an oven-proof dish and sprinkle with the crushed fennel seeds and black pepper
3. Shake the lemon juice, olive oil and stock/wine together and pour over the chicken and fennel
4. Bake for 30–35 minutes or until the chicken is cooked through

BAKED CHICKEN WITH OLIVES AND TOMATOES
Preparation time: 10 minutes
Cooking time: 35–40 minutes

3 medium potatoes
3–4 chicken breasts, cut into 3 or 4 slices
6–8 garlic cloves, peeled and sliced
1 red onion, sliced
200g cherry tomatoes, halved
½ cup kalamata olives
¼ cup fresh basil or oregano, chopped
1 tbsp lemon or lime juice
3–4 tbsp olive oil
1 tsp coarse black pepper

1. Preheat the oven to 190°C
2. Parboil the potatoes, then drain and cut into thick slices
3. Place the potatoes in the bottom of an oven-proof dish, top with the chicken and add the garlic, onion, tomatoes, olives and herbs

4. Shake the olive oil and lemon juice together, pour over the chicken and sprinkle with black pepper
5. Bake in the oven for 25–30 minutes or until the chicken is cooked through

BAKED LIME CHICKEN
Preparation time: 5 minutes
Cooking time: 30–35 minutes

3–4 chicken breasts, skinned
3 tbsp olive oil
1 tbsp grated fresh ginger
1 cup fresh coriander, chopped
zest and juice of 2 limes or 1 large lemon

1. Preheat the oven to 190°C
2. Put the chicken into an oven-proof baking dish
3. Shake the olive oil, ginger, coriander, lime zest and juice together and pour over the chicken, stir to coat the chicken in the marinade and leave for at least an hour
4. Bake for 30–35 minutes or until the chicken is cooked through

Alternatively, remove the chicken from the marinade and grill for 10–15 minutes, turning occasionally until the chicken is just cooked.

CHICKEN CURRY
Preparation time: 10 minutes
Cooking time: 30–40 minutes

2 tbsp vegetable oil
1 onion, peeled and chopped
4 garlic cloves, crushed
1 tbsp grated fresh ginger
2 tbsp curry powder
1 tsp cayenne pepper
200ml coconut milk or cream
2 tbsp desiccated coconut
1 cup chicken or vegetable stock
4 chicken breasts or thighs, skinned, boned and diced
60g green beans, sliced

1 × 120g tin bamboo shoots
1 cup frozen peas
1 cup frozen corn
1 cup bean sprouts
½ cup fresh coriander, chopped

1. Heat the vegetable oil and fry the onion for 3–4 minutes, then add the garlic, ginger, curry powder and cayenne pepper and continue to fry for another 1–2 minutes
2. Add the coconut milk, desiccated coconut and stock, and simmer briskly, stirring occasionally until the curry sauce has reduced
3. Add the chicken and beans and continue to simmer for 7–8 minutes or until the chicken is nearly cooked through, then add the bamboo shoots, peas and corn and continue to cook for another 2–3 minutes until the peas and corn are heated through
4. Just before serving stir through the bean sprouts and coriander

CHICKEN TERIYAKI
Preparation time: 2 minutes plus 2 hours to marinate
Cooking time: 15–20 minutes

2 tbsp olive oil
2 tbsp mirin or Chinese cooking wine
4 tbsp light soya sauce
4 chicken breasts, skinned

1. Shake the olive oil, mirin and soya sauce together, pour over the chicken breasts and leave to marinate for about 2 hours
2. Add the chicken, with the marinade, to a frying pan and cook for about 15–20 minutes, or until the chicken is cooked through, turning occasionally
3. Serve the chicken onto 4 plates and pour over a little of the cooked sauce

CORIANDER CHICKEN
Preparation time: 5 minutes plus an hour or more to marinate
Cooking time: 10–15 minutes

1 cup fresh coriander leaves
¼ cup fresh mint leaves

1 green chilli
2–3 garlic cloves, peeled
2 tbsp lemon juice
¼ cup olive oil
4 chicken thighs, skinned and boned

1. Put the coriander, mint, chilli, garlic and lemon juice in a food processor and slowly add the olive oil until it forms a smooth paste (add a little more olive oil if necessary)
2. Put the chicken in a single layer in a dish, pour over the coriander paste and turn the chicken to ensure both sides are well coated, then leave to marinate for at least an hour
3. Grill the chicken until cooked through, turning once or twice (the time will vary slightly depending on the size of the thighs)

GARLIC CHICKEN CASSEROLE
Preparation time: 5 minutes
Cooking time: 50–60 minutes

12 baby new potatoes, scrubbed
6–8 chicken thighs, skinned and boned, and halved
12–16 garlic cloves, peeled
4–6 shallots, halved
4 sprigs thyme
12 sage leaves
1–2 tbsp olive oil
½ cup chicken stock
1 tbsp lemon juice
1 tsp ground black pepper

1. Preheat the oven to 190°C
2. Parboil the potatoes for about 10 minutes, then drain
3. Place the chicken thighs, garlic, shallots, potatoes, thyme and sage in an oven-proof casserole dish
4. Shake the olive oil, stock, lemon juice and black pepper together and pour over the chicken
5. Cover and cook in the oven for 30–35 minutes, then remove the lid and cook for another 10–15 minutes (if you use chicken legs and/or thighs with the bone in, this dish will take slightly longer to cook)

GRILLED CHICKEN WITH OLIVE TAPENADE
Preparation time: 5 minutes
Cooking time: 5–10 minutes

2 tbsp olive oil
3–4 boned chicken thighs or breasts, skinned and cut into strips
2–3 tbsp olive tapenade (page 233)

1. Heat the olive oil and sauté the chicken for about 5 minutes until they are cooked through, stirring occasionally
2. Add the olive tapenade, stir to mix through the olive oil and cook for another 1–2 minutes until it is heated through

GRILLED GARLIC CHICKEN
Preparation time: 5 minutes plus 2 hours to marinate
Cooking time: 15–20 minutes

4–5 large garlic cloves, crushed
1 tsp coarse black pepper
2 tbsp fish sauce
¼ tsp palm or brown sugar
4 chicken thighs

1. Mix the garlic, pepper, fish sauce and sugar together, pour over the chicken and stir to make sure the chicken is well covered, then leave to marinate for at least 2 hours
2. Grill the chicken for about 15–20 minutes, turning regularly

GRILLED PEPPER CHICKEN
Preparation time: 5 minutes plus 30 minutes to marinate
Cooking time: 10–15 minutes

3–4 garlic cloves, crushed
2 tsp grated fresh ginger
1 tbsp cracked black pepper
2 tbsp light soya sauce
4 small chicken breasts, skinned

1. Mix together the garlic, ginger, black pepper and soya sauce, pour over the chicken and leave it to marinate for at least 30 minutes

2. Remove the chicken from the marinade and grill until it is just cooked through (about 10–15 minutes), turning occasionally
3. Heat any remaining marinade and pour over the chicken

ROAST CHICKEN LEGS WITH GINGER
Preparation time: 5 minutes plus 3 hours to marinate
Cooking time: 45–50 minutes

1 tbsp minced ginger
1 tbsp lemon juice
1 tbsp mirin
1 tbsp light soya sauce
4 whole chicken legs, skinned

1. Shake the ginger, lemon juice, mirin and soya sauce together
2. Place the chicken legs in an oven-proof dish, pour the marinade over them and leave for at least 3 hours
3. Roast the chicken at 200°C in the oven for approximately 45–50 minutes (or until no blood oozes from the chicken legs if you pierce them with a skewer)

SPICY CHICKEN AND MIXED PEPPER TORTILLAS
Preparation time: 15 minutes plus 30 minutes to marinate
Cooking time: 20 minutes

1 avocado
2 tsp lemon juice
1 tsp cayenne pepper
1 tsp ground cumin
1 tsp ground coriander
2–3 tbsp olive oil
2–3 chicken breasts, sliced
2 red peppers, seeded and cut into slices
2 green peppers, seeded and cut into slices
1 large onion, sliced
2 tsp balsamic vinegar
8 tortillas
2 tbsp hummus (page 234)
3 vine-ripened tomatoes, sliced
¼ cup fresh coriander, chopped

1. Mix together the dry spices, 1 tablespoon of the olive oil and the remaining lemon juice in a nonmetallic bowl
2. Add the chicken and stir to ensure the slices are well coated with the spices, then leave to marinate for at least 30 minutes
3. Put the peppers and onion in a frying pan with the remaining olive oil and the balsamic vinegar, toss to ensure the peppers are well coated in the oil and sauté for about 10–15 minutes until they are soft
4. While the peppers are cooking, in a separate pan, fry the chicken pieces in the marinade for about 5–6 minutes until they are just cooked
5. Sprinkle the tortillas with a little water, wrap them in foil and put them into a preheated 150° oven for about 5 minutes to heat them through
6. Peel, stone and slice the avocado and toss in a little lemon juice
7. To serve, place a tortilla on a plate, spread it with some hummus, put some grilled peppers down the centre, then a few pieces of the chicken, and top with a few tomato and avocado slices and some fresh coriander
8. Roll up the tortilla, folding in one end, and serve

STIR-FRIED CHICKEN AND MUSHROOMS WITH NOODLES
Preparation time: 5–10 minutes plus 30 minutes to marinate
Cooking time: 8–10 minutes

1 tbsp grated fresh ginger
2 tbsp mirin
2 tbsp light soya sauce
3–4 chicken thighs, skinned and sliced
400g soba noodles
2 tbsp olive oil
3–4 garlic cloves, sliced
2 tsp sweet chilli sauce
4–6 spring onions, sliced
150g fresh oyster mushrooms, halved
180g fresh baby sweet corn, halved
350g choi sum, cut into 3–4 pieces
1 tbsp oyster sauce
fresh coriander

1. Stir together the ginger, mirin and soya sauce in a nonmetallic bowl, add the chicken and stir to coat it in the marinade, then leave for at least half an hour
2. Cook the noodles according to the instructions on the packet, then drain and run under cold water
3. Heat the oil in a wok, remove the chicken from the marinade, reserving the marinade, and stir-fry the chicken for 2–3 minutes until just cooked through, then remove from the pan and keep warm
4. Add the garlic, chilli sauce and spring onions to the pan and stir-fry for 1 minute, then add the mushrooms and sweet corn and continue to stir-fry for another minute
5. Return the chicken to the pan, add the choi sum and noodles, stir through the oyster sauce and remaining marinade and continue to stir-fry for another 1–2 minutes until the choi sum has wilted and the noodles are heated through
6. Serve garnished with fresh coriander

STIR-FRIED CHICKEN WITH BEAN SPROUTS AND RED PEPPER
Preparation time: 15 minutes
Cooking time: 10–12 minutes

2 tbsp olive oil
3–4 garlic cloves, finely sliced
1 tbsp grated fresh ginger
1 tsp chilli sambal or 1 red chilli, finely sliced
2–3 boned chicken thighs, skinned and thinly sliced
2–3 celery stalks, sliced
1 red pepper, seeded and sliced
4–5 chestnut mushrooms, sliced
2 tbsp soya sauce
2 tbsp Chinese rice wine
3 cups bean sprouts
12–16 mangetout, halved
1 tbsp sesame oil
fresh coriander, chopped

1. Heat the olive oil in a frying pan or wok, add the garlic, ginger and chilli and stir-fry for 1 minute, then add the chicken pieces and stir-fry until it has just cooked through (approximately 3–4 minutes), then remove the chicken from the pan and keep warm

2. Add the celery, red pepper and mushrooms to the pan, stir to coat in the oil then add the soya sauce and rice wine and stir-fry briskly for 2–3 minutes, stirring occasionally
3. Add the bean sprouts, mangetout, chicken and sesame oil to the pan and continue to stir-fry for another 1–2 minutes until the vegetables are tender but still crisp; serve garnished with fresh coriander

STIR-FRIED CHICKEN WITH MANGETOUT
Preparation time: 5–10 minutes
Cooking time: 6–8 minutes

2 tbsp olive oil
3–4 chicken thighs, skinned and sliced
3–4 garlic cloves, sliced
1 tbsp grated fresh ginger
2 tsp sweet chilli sauce
4–6 spring onions, sliced
100g fresh oyster mushrooms, halved
200g mangetout, trimmed and cut in half
2 tbsp oyster sauce
1 tbsp light soya sauce
fresh coriander

1. Heat the olive oil in a wok and stir-fry the chicken for 3–4 minutes until it is just cooked through, then remove from the pan and keep warm
2. Add the garlic, ginger, chilli sauce and spring onions and stir-fry for 1 minute, then add the mushrooms and mangetout and continue to stir-fry for another minute
3. Return the chicken to the pan, add the oyster sauce, soya sauce and a dash of water and continue to stir-fry for another 1–2 minutes; serve garnished with fresh coriander

STIR-FRIED CHICKEN WITH MIXED PEPPERS
Preparation time: 10 minutes plus 1 hour to marinate
Cooking time: 10–12 minutes

4–5 garlic cloves, crushed
1 tbsp fresh ginger, grated

2 tbsp coarse black pepper
2–3 tbsp olive oil
4–6 boned chicken thighs, skinned and sliced
1 red onion, sliced
1 red pepper, seeded and sliced
1 green pepper, seeded and sliced
1–2 green or red chillies
1 cup fresh coriander, chopped

1. Mix together the garlic, ginger, black pepper and olive oil, pour over the chicken and marinate for at least 1 hour
2. Heat a wok or frying pan, add the chicken and marinade, and cook for 3–4 minutes until the chicken is just cooked, then remove the chicken from the pan and keep warm
3. Add the onion, peppers and chilli to the pan and sauté for 3–4 minutes, add a little water, cover and cook over a medium heat for another 5–6 minutes until the vegetables are cooked through
4. Return the chicken to the pan and heat through
5. Serve garnished with coriander

DUCK

SPICED DUCK BREAST WITH BROCCOLI
Preparation time: 5 minutes plus overnight to marinate
Cooking time: 15 minutes

2 tbsp olive oil
1 tbsp lemon juice
3–4 garlic cloves, crushed
1 tbsp grated ginger
½ tsp ground coriander
½ tsp ground cumin
½ tsp cayenne pepper
2–3 duck breasts, skinned and sliced
1 cup chicken or vegetable stock
3 star anise
1 cinnamon stick
½ red chilli, sliced
200g soft-stem broccoli

1 cup oyster mushrooms, halved
4 spring onions, sliced
60g mangetout
2 cups baby spinach leaves
1 cup bean sprouts
1 tbsp soya sauce
½ cup fresh coriander

1. Mix together the olive oil, lemon juice, garlic, ginger, corian-der, cumin and cayenne pepper
2. Add the sliced duck breast, stir to ensure it is coated in the spice mix and leave to marinate for at least 2 hours, or preferably overnight
3. Put the duck with the marinade in a frying pan and cook for about 5 minutes or until the duck is cooked through, then remove from the pan and keep warm
4. In a separate pan, heat the stock with the star anise, cinnamon stick and chilli and simmer for about 10 minutes, then remove the star anise and cinnamon stick
5. Add the broccoli and mushrooms to the stock and simmer for 2 minutes, then add the spring onions, mangetout, spinach and bean sprouts and simmer for another 1–2 minutes until the spinach is just wilted
6. Add the soya sauce and heat through
7. Divide the duck between four bowls, top with the vegetables and stock and garnish with fresh coriander

STIR-FRIED DUCK WITH PEPPERS AND NOODLES
Preparation time: 5 minutes
Cooking time: 15 minutes

250g fresh egg noodles
2 tbsp olive oil
2 duck breasts, skin removed and cut into strips
3 garlic cloves, sliced
1 tbsp grated fresh ginger
2 red chillies, sliced
1 tsp cracked black pepper
1 red pepper, sliced
1 green pepper, sliced

4–6 spring onions, sliced
2 tsp soya sauce
½ cup fresh coriander

1. Cook the noodles in plenty of boiling water according to the instructions on the packet, then drain and keep warm
2. Heat the olive oil in a wok or large frying pan and fry the duck strips for about 3–4 minutes until they are cooked through, then remove them from the pan and keep warm
3. Add the garlic, ginger, chillies and black pepper to the pan and stir-fry briefly, then add the red and green peppers and spring onions and continue to stir-fry for 2–3 minutes
4. Add the noodles to the pan and continue to stir-fry for another 3–4 minutes
5. Return the duck to the pan, toss to mix through the noodles and stir-fry for 1–2 minutes until they are heated through
6. Remove from the heat, stir through the fresh coriander and sprinkle with soya sauce

MEAT, NOW AND THEN

LAMB

PORK

Grilled or roast organic lamb, pork and occasionally beef and game, including rabbit and venison, are all acceptable in small quantities. If using minced meat, mince your own or get the butcher to freshly mince meat you have selected.

LAMB

MINCED LAMB BURGERS

Preparation time: 15 minutes plus 2 hours to marinate
Cooking time: 10–12 minutes

350g minced lamb
3–4 garlic cloves, finely chopped
1 red chilli, finely chopped
1 cup fresh coriander, finely chopped
¼ cup mint leaves, finely chopped
1 tbsp ground cumin
2 tsp paprika
1 tsp coarsely ground black pepper
2 spring onions, finely chopped
1 small egg

1. Put the lamb into a bowl and break it up with a fork, then add all the herbs and spices and the spring onions
2. Lightly whisk the egg and add it to the lamb, stir everything together to mix well, then cover and leave in the fridge for a couple of hours
3. Roll small balls of the mixture into slightly flattened burgers (it should make about 12) and fry in a griddle pan for about 5 minutes each side or until cooked through, turning them over carefully so they don't break up

MINCED LAMB SAMOSAS

This quantity makes about 50 small samosas. They are a little fiddly to make but are wonderful snacks. We find it easiest to make them over 2 days, cooking the lamb curry first and allowing it to cool as it is easier to handle when cold, completing the wrapping and frying the next day. The samosas can be kept frozen and warmed in the oven straight from the freezer.

Preparation time: filling 10–15 minutes; folding, approximately 30–40 minutes
Cooking time: filling 30–40 minutes; frying 15–20 minutes, reheating from frozen 10–15 minutes

2 tbsp olive oil
1 large onion, finely chopped
4–6 garlic cloves, finely chopped
1 tbsp grated fresh ginger
1–2 green chillies
2 tbsp curry powder
2 tsp cayenne pepper
500g minced lamb
½ cup water or stock
1 tbsp lemon juice
1½ cups frozen peas
1 cup fresh coriander, chopped
½ cup fresh mint, chopped
2 tsp garam masala
1 packet large spring roll pastry
vegetable oil for frying

1. Heat the olive oil in a wok or sauté pan and stir-fry the onion for 3–4 minutes, then add the garlic, ginger, chilli, curry powder and cayenne pepper and stir-fry for another minute
2. Add the lamb and stir-fry until it is well browned
3. Add the water and lemon juice and simmer, stirring occasionally, for 20–30 minutes until the lamb is tender and the liquid has been absorbed
4. Remove from the heat and stir through the peas, coriander, mint and garam masala and leave to cool
5. Thaw the pastry and cut the squares into three slices vertically (see diagram page 318)
6. Peel off a single piece of pastry, add a heaped teaspoonful of the meat mixture into the bottom right-hand corner of the pastry and keep folding the pastry until it forms a triangle (see diagram)
7. Heat the vegetable oil and shallow-fry the samosas a few at a time, until both sides are golden brown. Serve with sweet chilli dipping sauce

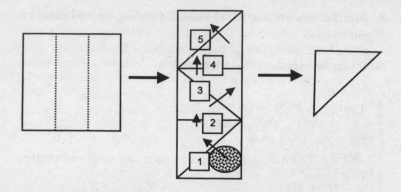

MOROCCAN LAMB MEATBALLS WITH SPICY TOMATO SAUCE
Preparation time: 15 minutes
Cooking time: 30 minutes

For the meatballs:
1 onion, peeled
½ cup flat-leaf parsley
½ cup fresh coriander
1 green chilli
1 tsp ground cumin
1 tsp ground cinnamon
350g minced lamb

For the sauce:
2 tbsp olive oil
1 onion, finely chopped
2 garlic cloves, crushed
1 red chilli, chopped
1 tsp ground cumin
1 tsp ground ginger
1 tsp paprika or cayenne pepper
400g canned tomatoes, chopped
2 tbsp chopped fresh flat-leaf parsley
2 tbsp chopped fresh coriander

1. Preheat the oven to 200°C
2. Process the onion, parsley, coriander and chilli in a food
   processor until finely chopped, then stir in the ground cumin
   and cinnamon and then add to the finely minced lamb

3. Roll the mixture into small balls, flatten slightly and place on an oiled baking tray and bake for 15 minutes until they become light brown in colour
4. While the meatballs are cooking, heat the olive oil in a frying pan and cook the onion for 4–5 minutes, then add the garlic, chilli and dry spices and sauté for another minute
5. Add the tomatoes and simmer for 15 minutes until the sauce has slightly thickened, then stir in the fresh parsley and coriander and cook for another 2 minutes
6. Add the meatballs to the tomato sauce and cook for another 10 minutes

RED CURRY LAMB CHOPS
Preparation time: 10 minutes plus 2 hours to marinate
Cooking time: 8–10 minutes

1–2 racks of lamb (about 8–10 ribs) or 8 small lamb chops or cutlets
2 tbsp Thai red curry paste (page 237)
1–2 tbsp olive oil
1–2 tbsp lemon juice

1. Cut the lamb racks into thin chops (this is most easily done when the meat is cold) and put them into a flat dish large enough to take them all in one layer
2. Mix together the red curry paste, olive oil and lemon juice, adjusting the quantity of olive oil and lemon juice so as to give a smooth, runny consistency
3. Pour the curry paste over the lamb chops and turn to ensure both sides of the chops are covered with the sauce; leave to marinate for at least 2 hours (preferably overnight)
4. Grill the chops for about 8–10 minutes, turning once or twice until they are done to your liking

SPICY ROAST LEG OF LAMB
Preparation time: 10 minutes plus overnight to marinate
Cooking time: 50–60 minutes plus 10 minutes standing time

¼ cup Thai red curry paste (page 237)
4–5 garlic cloves, crushed

2 tbsp lemon juice
4 tbsp olive oil
1 tbsp soya sauce
1 leg of lamb, butterflied

1. Preheat the oven to 190°C
2. Mix together the curry paste, garlic, lemon juice, olive oil and soya sauce
3. Make a few jabs in the lamb, put it into a large nonmetallic bowl, pour the curry sauce over it and leave to marinate overnight
4. Roast the lamb for approximately 50–60 minutes or until it is cooked to your liking
5. Leave to stand for 10 minutes before carving into thick slices

STIR-FRIED LAMB WITH GREEN PEPPER
Preparation time: 15 minutes
Cooking time: 15 minutes

500g lamb loin, sliced
3 tbsp olive oil
1 small red onion, sliced
3–4 garlic cloves, finely sliced
1 red chilli, finely sliced
2 green peppers, seeded and finely sliced
1 cup mangetout
1 tbsp sweet chilli sauce
3 tbsp fresh lime juice
2 tbsp fish sauce
½ cup fresh mint or basil leaves, chopped

1. Heat 1 tablespoon of the olive oil in a wok or frying pan and fry the lamb in batches for about 2 minutes or until browned, then remove the lamb and keep warm
2. Throw away any juices left in the pan, then add the remaining olive oil and stir-fry the onion for 3–4 minutes
3. Add the garlic and chilli and continue to fry for another minute, then add the green pepper and mangetout and continue to fry for 2–3 minutes
4. Return the lamb to the pan, add the chilli sauce, lime juice and fish sauce and stir-fry for another 2 minutes or until the lamb

is cooked through and the vegetables are soft, then stir through the mint leaves

PORK

MINCED PORK WITH GREEN BEANS
Preparation time: 3–4 minutes
Cooking time: 6–8 minutes

2 tbsp olive oil
4–5 garlic cloves, chopped
1 red chilli, sliced
1 tsp cayenne pepper
1 red pepper, sliced
400g green beans, cut into 3cm pieces
250g pork fillet, minced
1 cup water
1 tbsp fish sauce

1. Heat the olive oil and stir-fry the garlic, chilli and cayenne pepper for 30 seconds, add the red pepper, beans and pork and stir-fry for 2–3 minutes until the pork has changed colour
2. Add the water and fish sauce, cover the pan and cook until the beans are tender – about 3–4 minutes

MINCED PORK WITH NOODLES
Preparation time: 5 minutes
Cooking time: 6–8 minutes

250g thin egg noodles
2 tbsp olive oil
4–5 garlic cloves, minced
1 tbsp grated ginger
1–2 fresh large green chillies, finely chopped
500g pork fillet, minced
¼ cup light soya sauce
¼ cup water
2 tbsp mirin or Chinese cooking wine
6 spring onions
180g baby spinach leaves
100g mangetout

100g bean sprouts
¼ cup fresh mint, chopped
½ cup fresh coriander, chopped

1. Cook the noodles in a large saucepan of boiling water according to the instructions on the packet, then drain and keep warm
2. While the noodles are cooking, heat the olive oil in a wok and stir-fry the garlic, ginger and chillies for about a minute
3. Add the pork and continue to stir-fry, stirring until all the pork has changed colour
4. Add the soya sauce, water and mirin and heat through
5. Add the spring onions, spinach, mangetout, bean sprouts and mint, cover and continue to stir-fry until the spinach is just wilted, then stir through the coriander
6. Divide the noodles among four plates and top with the pork and vegetables

MINCED PORK WITH WATER CHESTNUTS
Preparation time: 15 minutes (if mincing your own pork)
Cooking time: 5 minutes

1 tbsp vegetable oil
2–3 garlic cloves, chopped
1 tbsp grated fresh ginger
1 tsp chilli sambal
6 spring onions, finely sliced
400g pork loin, minced
100g water chestnuts, chopped
1 tbsp soya sauce
1 tbsp sesame oil
1 tbsp plum sauce
1 cup fresh coriander, chopped

1. Heat the vegetable oil and stir-fry the garlic, ginger, chilli sambal and spring onions for 1 minute, then add the minced pork and continue to stir-fry for another 3–4 minutes until the pork has changed colour
2. Add the water chestnuts, soya sauce, sesame oil and plum sauce, and continue to sauté for another minute to heat through, then stir through the coriander

PORK LARB
Preparation time: 10 minutes
Cooking time: 8–10 minutes

3 tbsp chicken stock
3 garlic cloves, crushed
1 red chilli, finely sliced
¼ tsp palm sugar
250g minced pork
250g green beans, halved
1 red onion, finely sliced
2–3 spring onions, finely sliced
1 cup coriander, chopped
14 cup mint leaves, chopped
3 tbsp lime juice
1 tbsp fish sauce

1. Heat the stock in a frying pan, add the garlic, chilli and sugar and simmer for 1 minute, then add the pork and stir-fry until it changes colour
2. Add the green beans, cover the pan and cook for about 5 minutes until the beans are tender (they should still be crunchy)
3. Remove from the heat and stir through the red onion, spring onions, coriander, mint, lime juice and fish sauce (stir through a little chilli sambal if not spicy enough)

STIR-FRIED PORK TENDERLOIN AND MIXED VEGETABLES
Preparation time: 10 minutes plus 15 minutes to marinate
Cooking time: 10 minutes

3–4 garlic cloves
1 tbsp grated fresh ginger
1 red chilli, sliced
2 tbsp light soya sauce
1 tbsp Chinese cooking wine
350g pork tenderloin fillet, thinly sliced
2 tbsp olive oil
1 red onion, sliced
200g soft-stemmed broccoli, sliced
1 medium zucchini, sliced

8–10 spring onions, sliced
12 baby mushrooms
16–20 mangetout
2 stalks celery, thickly sliced
¼ cup water
1 tbsp oyster sauce
1 tbsp sesame oil

1. Shake the garlic, ginger, chilli, soya sauce and Chinese cooking wine together, pour over the sliced pork and leave to marinate for 15 minutes
2. Heat the olive oil in a large frying pan or wok and fry the onion for 2–3 minutes
3. Add the pork and marinade, and cook until all the pork has changed colour
4. Add the broccoli, zucchini, spring onions, mushrooms, mangetout and celery to the pan with a little water, cover and cook briskly for 2–3 minutes, then stir through the oyster sauce and sesame oil and continue to stir-fry until the vegetables are just cooked

THAI RED CURRY PORK WITH RICE NOODLES
Preparation time: 10 minutes
Cooking time: 10 minutes

450g rice vermicelli noodles
2 tbsp olive oil
350g pork fillet, thinly sliced
4 garlic cloves, crushed
1 red chilli, thinly sliced or 1 tsp chilli sambal
2 tbsp red curry paste (see page 237)
1 red pepper, sliced
6 spring onions, sliced
60g mangetout
2 tbsp fish sauce
1 tbsp fresh lime juice
100g baby spinach leaves

1. Put the noodles into a bowl, pour over boiling water and leave for approximately 5 minutes or cook according to the instructions on the packet, then drain and set aside

2. Heat the olive oil in a frying pan or wok and stir-fry the pork slices for 2–3 minutes until they are just cooked through, then remove them from the pan and keep warm
3. Add the garlic, chilli, red curry paste, red pepper, spring onions and mangetout and stir-fry for 2–3 minutes until the vegetables are soft
4. Return the pork to the pan and add the noodles, fish sauce, lime juice and spinach, and stir-fry until the spinach has just wilted

VERY EASY SWEET AND SOUR PORK
Preparation time: 15 minutes
Cooking time: 15 minutes

2 tbsp olive oil
350g pork fillet, thinly sliced
1 onion, sliced
4–5 garlic cloves, thinly sliced
1 red chilli or 1 tsp chilli sambal (or to taste)
4 tbsp tomato ketchup
2–3 tbsp rice vinegar
2 celery stalks, thickly sliced
1 red pepper, seeded and diced
8–12 baby sweet corn, cut in half
4–5 spring onions, coarsely sliced
fresh coriander

1. Heat the olive oil and stir-fry the pork slices for 3–4 minutes until they have changed colour, then remove the pork from the pan and keep warm
2. Add the onion to the pan and stir-fry for 2–3 minutes, then add the garlic, chilli, tomato ketchup and rice vinegar and continue to stir-fry for another minute
3. Add the celery, red pepper and sweet corn and continue to stir-fry for about 5 minutes until the vegetables are just cooked through (add a little water if the sauce is too thick)
4. Return the pork to the pan, add the spring onions and continue frying until the pork is heated through, then stir through the fresh coriander

Desserts

The best dessert is a plate of fresh fruit; however, here are some simple alternatives.

APRICOT TART
Preparation time: 5 minutes
Cooking time: 20 minutes

½ cup dark muscovado or molasses sugar
¼ cup water
grape-seed oil
8–10 apricots, halved and stoned
1 sheet puff pastry (dairy-free)

1. Preheat the oven to 200°C
2. Put the sugar and water in a small saucepan and simmer briskly until it becomes caramelised
3. Grease the bottom and sides of a nonstick baking tray with the grape-seed oil and pour in the caramel
4. Add the fruit, cut side down, ensuring the pieces are all close together, cover with the puff pastry and tuck the sides of the puff pastry inside the baking tray
5. Bake for about 20 minutes until the pastry has risen and is a lovely brown colour
6. Serve directly from the pan, or very carefully invert onto a serving plate that can catch any of the caramel

BAKED CUSTARD TART
Preparation time: 10 minutes
Cooking time: 60–70 minutes

1 cooked short-crust pastry case
1 egg white, lightly beaten
1 cup soya milk
1 cup soya cream
1 vanilla pod or a couple of drops of vanilla essence
3 tbsp unrefined cane caster sugar
2 eggs
2 egg yolks
Freshly grated nutmeg

1. Preheat the oven to 200°C
2. Brush the cooked pastry case with the beaten egg white and put into the oven for 5 minutes to seal the crust

3. Heat the soya milk and soya cream with the vanilla, add the sugar and stir until the sugar is dissolved, then strain if you have used a vanilla pod
4. Whisk the eggs and egg yolks together, then gradually add the soya milk and cream and stir gently to make the custard
5. Pour the custard into the pastry case and bake for 50–60 minutes until it has just set
6. When it is cooked, remove from the oven, grate nutmeg over the top and leave it to cool

BAKED PEACHES WITH AMARETTI BISCUITS
Preparation time: 5 minutes
Cooking time: 20–25 minutes

4 large peaches, halved and stoned
50g amaretti biscuits, crushed
⅓ cup Amaretto liqueur

1. Preheat the oven to 180°C
2. Put the peaches in a small baking tray, cut side up, put a spoonful of the crushed amaretti biscuits on top of each of the peaches, sprinkle with the liqueur and bake for about 20 minutes or until the peaches are well cooked through and soft

BANANA ICE CREAM
Preparation time: 5 minutes plus chilling time

400g bananas, peeled
½ cup unrefined cane caster sugar
½ cup soya cream
1 tbsp fresh lemon juice
2 tbsp dark rum (optional)

1. Purée the banana, sugar, cream and lemon juice together until smooth, stir in the rum, then freeze in a covered container or in an ice-cream maker

CARAMELISED MINTED ORANGES
Preparation time: 5–10 minutes
Cooking time: 15 minutes plus chilling time

¼ cup unrefined cane sugar
1 cup white wine

½ cup water
1 cinnamon stick
4 cloves
zest of one small lemon
4 oranges, peeled and sliced
2–3 tbsp finely chopped fresh mint

1. Put sugar, wine and water in a saucepan with the cinnamon, cloves and lemon zest, bring to a boil and simmer for 15 minutes
2. Remove the spices and pour the syrup over the oranges, sprinkle with the mint and chill in the refrigerator for at least 4 hours

CHOCOLATE SOUFFLÉ WITH RASPBERRIES
Preparation time: 5–10 minutes
Cooking time: 15 minutes

2 egg yolks
100g dark chocolate (non-dairy)
3 egg whites
¼ cup unrefined cane caster sugar
250g raspberries
soya cream

1. Preheat the oven to 180°C
2. Beat the egg yolks
3. Melt the chocolate in a bowl over a saucepan of simmering water, stirring until it is all melted and smooth, then remove from heat and stir into the egg yolks
4. Beat the egg whites until soft peaks form, then gradually add the sugar, beating continuously
5. Add the egg white to the chocolate mixture, stir to mix through, then spoon into soufflé dishes
6. Bake in the oven for about 10 minutes until they have risen and serve immediately with fresh raspberries and soya cream

GRAPEFRUIT AND CAMPARI SORBET
Preparation time: 5 minutes plus freezing time

2 cups pink or red fresh grapefruit juice
2 cups fresh orange juice

½ cup unrefined cane caster sugar
½ cup Campari

1. Mix all the ingredients together, stirring to dissolve the sugar
2. Process in an ice-cream maker or, if you don't have one, just put into the freezer

Variation: we often make this with fresh mandarin juice, which is very popular

GRILLED MANGO
Preparation time: 5 minutes
Cooking time: 8–10 minutes

2 large ripe mangoes
unrefined brown or molasses sugar
fresh lime juice

1. Cut the mango on either side of the stone
2. Cut a crisscross pattern into the top of each mango 'cheek', making sure not to cut through the skin
3. Sprinkle with lime juice and dust with a generous amount of brown sugar
4. Grill until soft and caramelised

GRILLED PINEAPPLE
Preparation time: 15 minutes
Cooking time: 15–20 minutes

1 pineapple
⅓ cup rum (optional)
¼ cup unrefined brown or molasses sugar

1. Choose a ripe pineapple, as they do not ripen once they have been picked
2. Cut the top and base off the pineapple, then peel it, removing all the black bits by cutting around the pineapple with 'v' shaped incisions
3. Cut into thick slices and remove the central core
4. Sprinkle with the sugar and rum and grill for about 15 minutes

INDIVIDUAL APPLE TARTS
Preparation time: 5 minutes
Cooking time: 10–15 minutes

1 sheet prepared puff pastry (non-dairy)
4 green apples, cored and sliced
1 tbsp unrefined brown sugar

1. Preheat the oven to 200°C
2. Cut the pastry into 4 squares, top with the apple slices and sprinkle with brown sugar
3. Bake for 10–15 minutes or until the pastry is puffed and golden

MIXED BERRY SALAD
Preparation time: 5 minutes plus 20 minutes marinating time

200g strawberries
1–2 tbsp unrefined cane sugar
juice of 1 lemon
200g raspberries
100g blackberries
200g blueberries

1. Cut the strawberries in half (or quarters if very large), then sprinkle over the sugar, pour over the lemon juice, stir carefully and leave to marinate for about 20 minutes
2. Just before serving, stir through the raspberries, blackberries and blueberries

Variation: instead of lemon juice use 1–2 tbsp of Cointreau or Drambuie

PEAR AND ALMOND TARTS
Preparation time: 1–2 minutes
Cooking time: 30–35 minutes

2 pears, peeled
1 tbsp fresh lemon juice
½ cup unrefined cane caster sugar
1 vanilla bean
1–2 sheets non-dairy puff pastry
100g marzipan
1 small egg, lightly beaten

1. Preheat the oven to 190°C
2. Cut the pears in half and toss in the lemon juice
3. Heat 1 cup of water in a saucepan, add the sugar and vanilla bean and simmer until the sugar has dissolved, then add the pears and simmer for about 10 minutes or until the pears are soft
4. Remove the pears from the pan, remove the cores and slice them lengthways, leaving the thin end whole, and spread to form a 'fan'
5. Cut the pastry into 4 circles, slightly larger than the pears, and put onto baking paper on a baking tray, place a slice of marzipan on each circle of pastry, top with a pear and lightly score the pastry around the edges, not cutting right through, then brush with the beaten egg
6. Cook for 20–25 minutes until the pastry has puffed

POACHED PEACHES WITH RASPBERRY COULIS
Preparation time: 10 minutes
Cooking time: 2–3 minutes

3–4 peaches, halved and stoned
200g fresh or frozen raspberries
1 tbsp unrefined cane caster sugar

1. Poach the peaches in a little water for 2–3 minutes, then take out of the water, remove the skins, slice and divide among serving plates
2. Purée the raspberries with the sugar in a blender and pour over the peaches

POACHED RED GRAPES
Preparation time: 1–2 minutes
Cooking time: 10 minutes

1 cup red grape juice or red wine
½ cup unrefined cane caster sugar
125g raisins
1 cinnamon stick
400g red grapes, washed and dried
1 tbsp lemon juice

1. Put the grape juice or red wine, sugar, raisins and cinnamon in a pan and simmer briskly for 5 minutes
2. Add the grapes and lemon juice and continue to simmer for another 5 minutes; remove the cinnamon stick before serving

POACHED STRAWBERRIES
Preparation time: 5 minutes
Cooking time: 5 minutes

2 cups very ripe strawberries, washed and halved
¼–½ cup fresh orange juice
2 tbsp unrefined caster sugar
1 tbsp Cointreau (optional)

1. Put all the ingredients into a saucepan and simmer gently until the berries are soft but still have some shape

RASPBERRY ICE CREAM
Preparation time: 5–10 minutes

200g fresh or frozen raspberries
1 tbsp fresh lemon juice
½ cup unrefined caster sugar
½ cup water
¼ cup soya cream
2 tbsp Kir or other liqueur (optional)

1. Purée the raspberries with the lemon juice, sugar and water until smooth
2. Stir the cream through the raspberries, then stir through the liqueur
3. Freeze in a covered container or in an ice-cream maker; soften slightly in the fridge before serving

RASPBERRY TRIFLE
Preparation time: 20–30 minutes plus cooling time
Cooking time: 5–6 minutes

1 cup soya milk and 1 cup soya cream
2–3 drops vanilla essence or 1 vanilla bean
1 tbsp grated orange peel

5 egg yolks
½ cup unrefined cane sugar
50g cornflour
1 packet vegetarian jelly crystals
130g amaretti biscuits or almond macaroons
2 tbsp Cointreau, Grand Marnier or sherry
225g fresh or frozen raspberries
½ cup soya cream
small block of dairy-free dark chocolate

1. Heat the soya milk and cream with the vanilla essence and orange peel until it begins to simmer, then remove from the heat
2. Beat together the egg yolks, sugar and cornflour until they become pale yellow and quite thick, then slowly add the heated soya milk, continuing to whisk until it is smooth
3. Return the mixture to the pan and cook over a moderate heat, stirring continuously, until it thickens and has just started to boil, then take off the heat and beat vigorously for 1 minute; pour through a coarse strainer and leave to cool
4. Pour boiling water on the jelly crystals and leave to cool, then put in the freezer, but remove before the jelly becomes solid
5. Put the amaretti biscuits into the bottom of a (preferably) glass bowl and pour the liqueur over them
6. Top with the raspberries then cover with the jelly – it should still be quite soft
7. Pour over the custard, cover and leave to chill until you are ready to serve
8. Just before serving pour over a layer of soya cream and grate over some dark chocolate

SOYA ICE CREAM
Preparation time: 15 minutes plus freezing time to
Cooking time: 5–6 minutes

2 medium eggs
2 egg yolks
¼ cup unrefined caster sugar
1 cup unsweetened soya milk
½ cup soya cream

1 tbsp grated orange peel
2 tbsp Cointreau (optional)

1. Beat the eggs, yolks and sugar together until they turn pale yellow in colour and form soft ribbons
2. Put the soya milk, soya cream and orange peel in a saucepan and bring to a gentle simmer, then add to the eggs, a little at a time, beating continuously, before returning to the saucepan and heating gently for 2–3 minutes
3. Stir through the Cointreau, allow to cool, then process in an ice-cream maker

> Tip: If you don't have an ice-cream maker, make a sorbet or even ice cream by freezing the mixture until it is almost set, then remove from the freezer and stir to break up the ice crystals and put back in the freezer until it sets.

TOFU ICE CREAM
Preparation time: 5 minutes plus freezing time

450g ripe bananas, peeled and sliced
1 cup fresh orange juice
150g soft tofu
2 tbsp honey

1. Purée all the ingredients together in a food processor
2. Put in the freezer for about 4 hours until frozen but not solid

WHITE WINE AND LEMON JELLY WITH POACHED GRAPES AND BLUEBERRIES
Preparation time: 5 minutes
Cooking time: 10 minutes plus chilling time

2 cups white wine
½ cup water
½ cup fresh lemon juice
3 tbsp lemon rind
2 cinnamon sticks
2 cloves
1 × 85g packet of vegetarian lemon-jelly crystals

2 cups fresh seedless red grapes
2 tbsp unrefined cane sugar
1 punnet blueberries
soya cream

1. Simmer the wine, water, lemon juice, lemon rind, cinnamon and cloves for about 5 minutes, then remove the spices
2. Put the jelly crystals into a bowl, pour the heated wine over them and stir to dissolve the crystals, then put in the fridge to set
3. Put the grapes in a small saucepan, sprinkle over the sugar and a little water, and poach for about 5 minutes, then remove from the heat and stir through the blueberries
4. Divide the fruit among serving bowls, add the jelly and top with soya cream

Index